THE PRINCIPLES
OF BIOMEDICAL
INSTRUMENTATION
A Beginner's Guide

D1444991

THE PRINCIPLES OF BIOMEDICAL INSTRUMENTATION
A Beginner's Guide

STANLEY A. RUBIN, M.D.
Associate Professor of Medicine
UCLA School of Medicine
Director, Cardiology Training Program
Cedars-Sinai Medical Center
Los Angeles, California

YEAR BOOK MEDICAL PUBLISHERS, INC.
Chicago • London

1 2 3 4 5 6 7 8 9 0 CY 91 90 89 88 87

Library of Congress Cataloging-in-Publication Data
Rubin, Stanley A.
    The Principles of Biomedical Instrumentation: A Beginner's Guide

    Bibliography: p.
    Includes index.
    1. Medical instruments and apparatus.   2. Biomedical engineering.   I. Title.
    R856.R83   1987   610'.28   86-24731
    ISBN 0-8151-7453-5

Sponsoring Editor: Richard H. Lampert
Manager, Copyediting Services: Frances M. Perveiler
Production Manager, Text and References/Periodicals: Etta Worthington
Proofroom Supervisor: Shirley E. Taylor

In loving memory of Nathan J. Rubin, and Irving R. Rose.
In honor of Ronnie, Joshua, and Rose.

Preface

The aim of this book is to present the basics of modern instrumentation so as to guide the novice user in becoming familiar with instruments, and to encourage the full and creative use of instruments for the collection and analysis of biological data.

This book originated at the suggestion of a student who attended my brief course on biomedical instrumentation. I give this course to cardiology fellows as they are preparing to enter the research aspects of their training. When he asked for a very basic textbook to supplement my lectures, and I couldn't cite one, he suggested that one be written based on material in the course. The book is the answer to that student's request. Technologically superior instruments are one of the bases of rapid advancements in biology and medicine. However, like the planetary explorers in the science fiction novel and movie *2001: A Space Odyssey*, the novice scientist stands in awe and sometimes confusion at the monolith of technology. This book moves the beginner beyond the paralysis that accompanies those primal feelings, by providing the essential information on the theory and operation of instruments.

The 11 chapters of the book can be partitioned into three sections: the principles, the hardware, and miscellany. The three chapters that compose the section on principles define the fundamentals of a biological signal, the rule governing measurements in general and how these relate to instrument errors, and classification and organization of instruments. A chapter on electrical principles and safety introduces this section. The section on hardware includes five chapters and is introduced by an overview of what defines an instrument and how multiple instruments are used together. Subsequent chapters discuss signal detectors, signal conditioners, recorders, and computers. The last section has three chapters on the use of instruments during data collection, repair and maintenance of instruments, and purchase of instruments.

I strongly advise the reader to review the early chapters that cover the principles before launching into the other two sections of the book. Both the concepts and the language used in these early chapters are key to maximizing the information content in the rest of the book.

In certain chapters on hardware, the reader will notice material that provides a certain amount of technical detail beyond what the beginner really needs to know. I make no apologies for this: the material is short, it's subject matter that you can master with a bit of tutoring, and you can always skip it if it's just too heavy. I always give you fair warning of what's ahead.

Single author textbooks on biomedical subjects are infrequent; and, despite the single name on the cover, you shouldn't suppose that the production of this book was unaided. In some ways, I can cite my mother and my piano teacher as the roots of this endeavor (see Chapter 2). More directly, I can cite a group of people who have had a substantial influence on my career: instrumentation engineers. These are the people who really understand the principles and the application of biomedical instrumentation, but who frequently travel in a different professional circle than the scientist or investigator. It has been my good fortune to have come into contact with a group of very capable instrumentation engineers, and to have been the beneficiary of an enormous amount of their time and perserverence. My good fortune began with my collaboration with Reginald Quilter at the National Institutes of Health, continued with Robert Battigan at the University of California, San Francisco, and concludes up to the present with David Mickle at Cedars-Sinai Medical Center. I want to pay special tribute to David for helping me prepare some of the material in this book, including the technical aspects of many of the chapters. Also at Cedars-Sinai, Simon Solingen has been very generous in his assistance. An unstated message in this book is that anyone who wants to know about or use biomedical instrumentation will reap benefit from a professional association with an instrumentation engineer.

There are a number of other people who I consider as unindicted co-conspirators in suggestions about, or actual preparation of, some of the material in this book. I consulted with Stanton A. Glantz, Ph.D., at the University of California, San Francisco, during the preparation of this book. In addition to the very useful guidance that he provided, Stan was also instrumental in recruiting the careful review and suggestions of Julian Hoffman, M.D., at the Cardiovascular Research Institute. At Cedars-Sinai, some of my colleagues made valuable contributions: Moraye Bear (Chapter 3) and Michael Shabot, M.D., and Brad Pollack (Chapter 8). The figures in the book brilliantly demonstrate the craft of the illustrator, Lance Laforteza, and the photographer, David Zagorski. I received technical assistance in the preparation of this book from my research associate, Tom Nusbickel, and my secretary, Beverly Yoshioka.

The support, encouragement, and understanding of my colleagues and family have sustained me during the preparation of this book. The calm reassurance, persistence and valuable insight of my Editor at Year Book, Richard Lampert, has been an important source of encouragement over the months of preparation of this book. I want to thank my boss, H.J.C. Swan, M.D., Ph.D, Director of Cardiology at Cedars-Sinai, for permitting me the time and freedom to undertake this project, and the faculty of the Division for tolerating me during my fits of self-indulgence. Finally, my family's encouragement and solace that accompanied the creation of this book, despite my erratic behavior, allowed me to bring this effort to a finality.

STANLEY A. RUBIN, M.D.

Contents

Electrical Safety and Instrument Hazards

Electrical safety and instrument hazards are a primary consideration in the use of instrumentation, not a final one. For that reason, this chapter appears at the front of this book. Don't read further, and certainly don't use any instruments, until you understand the principles of safety.

WHAT YOU NEED TO KNOW

1. No person should ever be jeopardized because of the lack of safety considerations. At particular risk is a patient or a subject (in an experiment). Other personnel, including the scientist, may also be at risk.

2. Electrical shock hazards are a major problem in the use of instrumentation. A thorough understanding of the principles of electricity and electrical power is needed to appreciate and reduce this hazard.

3. Electrical safety comes down to limiting the amount of current that passes through the body and especially through the heart or another vital organ system to extremely small values (a few microamps).

4. Other safety hazards exist that are dependent on the type of instrumentation or support equipment in use. These could include, for example, the inappropriate or inadvertent use of an instrument or the abnormal electrical, mechanical, or radiation function of an instrument.

Who Is at Risk

Any injury or death caused by instrumentation is unacceptable. The greatest hazard exists to the patient or subject who is linked to instrumentation for purposes of clinical monitoring or scientific study. Their hazard is greatly increased for a few reasons. First, they may not be in a position to recognize and ward off noxious events because their mobility or sensorium is impaired, either as a result of their illness or because of a medical procedure (consider the anesthetized patient). Second, the presence of multiple instrument connections and pieces of equipment greatly increases the opportunity for introducing electrical currents through a patient's body (see below). Third, monitoring equipment that breaches the skin (e.g., catheters) or reduces the normal resistance of the skin to the flow of electrical current (electrodes or moist/wet environments) greatly increases the electrical safety hazard.

Nonpatient personnel are also at risk for electrical injury, although the amount of electrical current that poses a hazard for them may be considerably larger than the threshold level for a patient. Of course, this higher level is of even greater hazard to a patient. Quantitation of shock level is described later in this chapter.

The number of accidents that involve instrumentation is large, and probably is underreported because of lack of careful investigation as to the cause of an injury (especially sudden death in ill patients). This is due to a failure to recognize the types of injuries that can be caused by instruments, and to the fear of reprisals or litigation in response to such a report.

Because of the current state of the art in the understanding of instrument safety, and because of the application of safety devices and safety maintenance, instrument hazards could be greatly reduced. Instrument users are the current weak link in the chain of instrument safety when there is improper attention to details of instrument inspection, maintenance, and application.

Principles of Electricity

The Electrical Circuit

A circuit is made of physical devices capable of conducting electricity. A circuit is capable of carrying current when it is physically complete and closed (in continuity). A circuit actually carries current when a voltage potential exists across two points in the circuit. The physical elements of the circuit must include conductors—materials capable of carrying current. Surprisingly, humans are made of conductive materials.

Voltage

Current flows because of a potential difference (E), the same way that water flows over and through a dam because of a gravitational difference between the top and the bottom of the waterfall (Fig 1–1). The unit of potential difference is the volt (V), and sources of electricity (whether at the wall socket, from a battery, or as part of an instrument) are, in part, rated by their voltage—that is, how much potential difference they can supply. Voltage sources are also characterized by the manner in which they generate the voltage (Fig 1–2): either cyclically

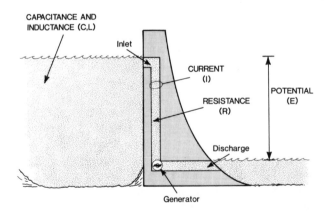

FIG 1–1.
The physical properties of a dam are a hydraulic analogy of electricity. The potential energy of the height of the water of the lake behind the dam in reference to the outlet of the dam is equivalent to an electrical potential (E). The flow of water through the dam is equivalent to that of current flow through a circuit (I). The loss of energy encountered by the flow of water through the dam is equivalent to resistance in an electrical circuit (R). The storage of the body of water in the lake behind the dam is equivalent to capacitance (C) and inductance (L) in an electrical circuit. The practical equivalence of the two can be demonstrated by inserting a generator in the dam: electrical power can then be produced from hydraulic power.

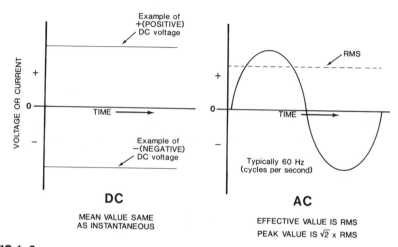

FIG 1–2.

Voltage and current are produced at constant levels *(DC)*, or cyclically *(AC)*. Batteries and power supplies within instruments typically produce DC. With respect to a reference level, DC voltage can be either positive or negative. Power available at the wall outlet generated by municipal power companies is almost always AC in the United States. With respect to a reference level, AC voltage swings between positive and negative values. For many purposes, it is convenient to express AC voltage and current levels as the effective equivalent of DC through the calculation of root mean square (RMS) values.

(sinusoidally alternating voltage at a specific frequency which therefore generates sinusoidally *alternating current,* or AC) or steady-state (direct voltage which therefore generates *direct current,* or DC).

Municipal power supplies in most of the world, including the United States, the United Kingdom, Europe, and Japan, are typically AC, but voltage potential and frequency may vary. Typically, line voltage at a wall outlet in the United States will be 60 Hz frequency, 110 VAC (with a range from 105 to 125 VAC) and less commonly (in the home or office) 220 VAC. However, most electrical and electronic equipment requires DC. Therefore, a large part of support equipment either inside or outside the instrument cabinet will be devoted to taking the AC voltage available at the power outlet (so-called line voltage) and converting it into DC and also perhaps altering its potential difference to a more suitable level. In a small instrument, the power supply (the device that alters line voltage) could well be rated at an input of 110 VAC and an output of 24 VDC. The power supply of a large instrument that requires high voltage for operation (such as a TV set or an x-ray tube) could be rated at an input of 110, 220, or 440 VAC and an output of 24,000 VDC (24 kilovolts, or kV).

Current

Charge (Q) is the mass of electricity, which is analogous to the mass of water in the lake of the dam. The unit of charge is the coulomb, which is 6.25×10^{18} electrons. Current (I) is the amount of electrical charge per unit time that flows in response to the potential difference (voltage), the same as the amount of water per unit time that flows over and through the dam (see Fig 1–1). The unit of current is the ampere or amp (A), which is a current flow of one coulomb per second. Electrical supplies are also, in part, rated by their amperage *capacity*—that is, the maximum current that they can deliver. Because of considerations related to the practical use and construction of wiring, the typical line current at a household outlet may be limited to 15 or 20 A by a special type of resistor called a fuse or by a circuit breaker (see below). A power supply for a small instrument may have a current capacity of 0.2 A (200 milliamps, or mA). A power supply for a very large piece of equipment could be rated at 1,000 A. When the current flow is AC or DC the accompanying voltage potential is the same specification.

Current Density

Current density is the ratio of the current flow to the area over which the current flows (Fig 1–3). Current density can change with either a change of current flow, or a change of area over which the current flows. This has extremely important implications for what ef-

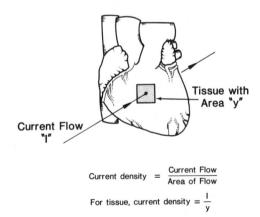

$$\text{Current density} = \frac{\text{Current Flow}}{\text{Area of Flow}}$$

$$\text{For tissue, current density} = \frac{I}{y}$$

FIG 1–3.
Many biologic effects of electricity—especially electrical shock—are determined by current density, which is the amount of current flow per unit of tissue area over which the current flows.

fect electricity has on biologic tissue, including shock hazard and damage to biologic tissue: the higher the current density, the more likely is the biologic effect.

Energy Dissipation and Storage

Resistance (R)—and its inverse, conductance—is the dissipative property of the electrical circuit, which is analogous to the energy loss (friction) as the water flows over and through the dam and as the molecules of water slide past one another in a viscous and turbulent manner (see Fig 1–1). Mechanical and electrical friction generates heat, and this can be used to good purpose in the creation of a resistance element that heats and then breaks if the flow of current is too large—the fuse.

Resistance is a basic property of all conductors and semiconductors, that is, materials capable of carrying current. Nonconductive materials (also called electrical insulators) have a very large resistance. The type of material through which the current will flow, its cross-sectional area, its length, and its temperature all determine the resistance—the smaller the cross-section, the longer the length, and the higher the temperature, the greater the resistance for any type material. The unit of resistance is the ohm (Ω), while the unit of conductance (1/resistance) is the mho.

Capacitance (C) and inductance (L) are the properties of circuit elements to store electrical energy, which is analogous to the storage of water in the lake behind the dam (see Fig 1–1). Capacitors store charge in an electrostatic field, while inductors store voltage in a magnetic field. The equivalent mechanical analogy of the capacitor is the potential energy stored by the lake as a result of its height above the outlet of the dam; the mechanical analogy of the inductor is the mass or inertiance of the body of water stored in the lake.

Capacitors consist of two conductor surfaces separated by a nonconductor. Capacitors either increase or decrease their charge in response to a respective increase or decrease of electrical potential. The unit of capacitance is the farad (F). They tend to pass AC, but block DC. Inductors consist of a multicoiled strand of conductor material (usually wire). Inductors increase or decrease their potential in response to a respective increase or decrease of current flow. The unit of inductance is the henry (H). They tend to pass DC, but block AC. Some electrical components are purposely designed to store energy. However, even when not purposely designed to store energy, the physical shape and material of construction of components, as in the case of an electrical instrument, may cause objects to act as inadvertent energy storage devices. As we will see below, this can cause an unexpected shock hazard.

Relationships Among Voltage, Current, and Resistance

Voltage and current values of DC power supplies are usually considered as constant over time, and therefore mean or average values are specified. Because the magnitude of AC is always changing, knowledge of instantaneous values is relatively unimportant compared to overall effect. Effective values of AC voltage and current are defined by equivalence to that which would be produced in a DC circuit for the same resistance. This effective value is called the root mean square, or RMS, value (see Fig 1–2).

In simplest form (and only appropriate for electrical power circuits) the voltage, current, and resistance are linearly related by Ohm's law, which allows calculation of one of the variables based on knowledge of the other two. The relationship can be conveniently demonstrated in the accompanying diagram (Fig 1–4). The values calculated from this relationship use mean values for DC and RMS values for AC. For example, an electrical heater on a 110 V circuit could have a resistance of 12 ohms, and therefore draw about 9.0 A of current. The total dissipative properties of the circuit are dependent on both the resistance (the dissipative property of resistors in a DC or AC circuit) and the reactance (the dissipative property of capacitors and inductors in an AC circuit). This is called impedance (Z). The relationships expressed in Ohm's law are the same, but the value of Z is substituted in place of R.

Energy is the work done, and is expressed as watt × second or its equivalent, the joule (J). Power is the rate of doing work, or the energy consumed per unit time in the electric circuit, and is expressed in watts (W). The linear relationship between power, current, and voltage is shown in the accompanying diagram (see Fig 1–4). Again, the values calculated from this relationship use mean values for DC and RMS values for AC. For example, the heater cited above on a 110 V circuit, which draws 9.0 A, would consume almost 1,000 W of power.

Electrical components that have the properties of resistance, capac-

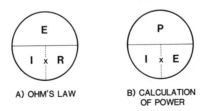

A) OHM'S LAW   B) CALCULATION
                         OF POWER

FIG 1–4.
Relationship among variables in Ohm's law *(left)* and power calculation *(right)*. In order to use, place a finger over the variable to be calculated, and obey the mathematical operation inferred by the diagram.

itance, and inductance are called resistors, capacitors, and inductors, respectively. When more than one physical component is used in a circuit they may be arranged by connecting one to another "head" to "tail" (elements connected in *series*), side by side with all "heads" connected and all "tails" connected (elements arranged in *parallel*), or a combination of multiple variations on the above (elements arranged in *series-parallel*). For elements arranged in series, current flow is equal through each element, and voltage is dependent on Ohm's law for each device. For elements arranged in parallel, voltage is equal across each element, and current flow is dependent on Ohm's law for each device. Power consumption for each circuit element is still calculated as the product of its current flow and voltage.

Electronics

Most instrumentation includes electronic components. The distinction between electrical power and electronics is tenuous. As an expression of this difference, a member of the electrical maintenance department once told an instrumentation engineer, "I take care of the thick wires, and you take care of the thin ones." However, life is not so simple. We will allude to one type of electronic component, the operational amplifier, in chapter 6.

Instruments That Measure Electrical Characteristics

Increasingly sophisticated instrumentation is available to measure and define electrical characteristics of both electrical power (the subject of the above material) and electronics (the subject of much of the remainder of this book). These test instruments in and of themselves are subject to the same principles of instrumentation described in the remainder of the book. The test instruments that are frequently used include the voltmeter, the volt-ohm-ammeter (VOM), and the oscilloscope. One of these devices should be present in each laboratory, and the investigator should be thoroughly familiar with their function. Clinical engineering departments and instrumentation engineers will have additional sophisticated test instruments.

Voltmeter.—This device observes electrical voltage and displays that value to the user in the form of a scale or digital display. The most versatile form of this instrument includes options for measuring AC or DC voltage, and different scales to optimize the reading capability of large and small voltages. Because DC voltage is unchanging or slowly changing, the voltmeter reports the actual level of voltage. Because AC voltage is constantly changing, and because meters and displays don't have the capability of reporting rapidly changing signals (see chapter 7) the value reported by the instrument in the AC mode is RMS. The voltmeter is especially useful in the setup and calibration of instrumentation (chapter 9).

VOM.—This is a multitalented display device that includes all the functions of the voltmeter as well as the capabilities for measuring resistance and current. For optimal use, each function will have a set of ranges to allow the measurement of large and small values. The VOM is essential for troubleshooting of instrumentation problems (chapter 10).

Oscilloscope.—This is, in essence, a voltmeter in which a simple meter or visual display has been replaced with a TV screen. The utility of this simple difference should not be underestimated. On the screen, the voltage level is observed on the "y" or vertical axis; the "x" or horizontal axis can be used for two purposes. First, the "x" axis can be a time scale that can be swept once across the screen to "freeze" an action, or repetitively to allow a continuous update of the voltage. Second, the display of the oscilloscope can be used to compare the level of two voltages simultaneously by also using the "x" axis as a scale of voltage. Timing can be made implicit by allowing the dual voltage readings to be displayed continuously on the screen. This test instrument is enormously valuable for observing voltages that are rapidly changing. It is widely used in instrument calibration, repair, and maintenance. It is also invaluable throughout the different phases of preparing for and acquiring data from signals, because it allows the investigator to see moment to moment changes of signal level.

Principles of Electrical Hazards

General Concepts of Electrical Shock

A potential for an electrical hazard exists whenever the body simultaneously contacts a higher and lower source of voltage potential and therefore completes a circuit that allows the flow of current through the body. The subtleties of this circuit are numerous and convoluted. A major hazard or threat to life exists when a large amount of current passes through the body, or a critical current density is achieved in a vital organ system; usually that organ is the heart, and sometimes the brain.

The body has a finite (usually high) resistance and normally acts as a poor conductor. The usual limitation to current flow through the body is the resistance of dry skin, the usual contact point of an electrical instrument or device. Dry skin has a resistance of perhaps 10,000 to 100,000 ohms or more. If the skin completes a circuit with a source of 110 V, approximately 0.001 to 0.01 A (1 to 10 mA) would flow through the body.

Macroshock.—The effects of these *macroshocks* (shocks of ≥1 mA) would be noted by the conscious person (Fig 1–5). The pathway of current through the body largely would be determined by the points of contact between the body and the higher and lower voltage potential points. Because the body is a sac filled with a fluid of good conducting properties (electrolyte), the current flow *would not* be over the surface of the skin, but rather through a large volume and area of tissue. Therefore, the current density achieved in the vital organ systems of the body would be small. However, effects on and near the points of contact would be noted. This would range from skin discomfort up to and including contraction of the muscle groups of the section of the body touching the electrical source (muscle depolarization and tetanic contraction). This latter observation is the "can't let go" phenomenon frequently reported in electrical safety literature. Although prolonged contact on a small patch of skin by this amount of current might result in a limited thermal or muscle injury, no grave harm would be done.

Ventricular Fibrillation.—Now contrast this with two other situations that involve *reduced resistance* and/or *reduced volume and area* of

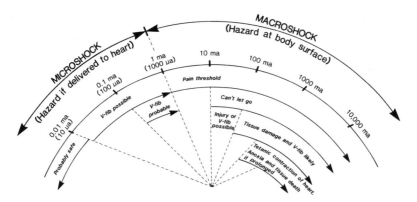

FIG 1–5.
Spectrum of shock hazard as a function of shock current. Shocks less than 1 mA are considered microshocks, and only are hazardous when delivered directly to tissue—especially the heart. Shocks greater than 1 mA are considered macroshocks and are hazardous even when delivered at the surface of the body.

tissue through which the current flows. If skin tissue is moistened (in a bathtub, swimming pool, or moist environment), or frankly contacted by an electrolyte solution or pad after removing the horny (outermost dead) layer of the epidermis, skin resistance can be greatly reduced, perhaps down to the range of 1,000 to 10,000 ohms. Current in response to 110 V potential applied to the skin would be approximately 10 to 100 mA. The latter figure may be high enough to cause pain, fainting, exhaustion, and mechanical injury. If the volume conductor includes the thorax, the size of this current flow and the achieved current density may be sufficient to cause ventricular fibrillation—a disorganized and ineffective cardiac contraction that quickly results in death unless corrected.

Currents from 100 to 1,000 mA are very likely to achieve this effect of ventricular fibrillation. Currents larger than 1,000 mA may occur when there is an even further reduction in skin resistance, or the application of a higher voltage. When passed through the body, such currents cause respiratory paralysis as long as they are maintained. Interestingly, these larger currents may not cause ventricular fibrillation, but rather ventricular tetany—a sustained but uniform contraction of the cardiac muscle. If removed before severe ischemia occurs, a regular respiratory and cardiac rhythm may be restored spontaneously. Even if no direct mechanical or thermal damage is apparent, cessation of cardiac or respiratory function for more than a few seconds will have grave consequences on organ systems with obligate oxygen metabolism such as the brain, and permanent neurologic sequelae or death may occur.

Microshock.—Smaller shocks, below 1 mA and labeled *microshocks,* may also have grave consequences when locally applied to the heart, even though they will not be felt (see Fig 1–5). If the pathway for these microshocks is through a device that breaches the skin and delivers the current in close proximity to the heart, microshocks may cause ventricular fibrillation. This device is usually an electrode catheter used for electrophysiologic diagnosis or therapy of cardiac arrhythmias. However, hollow catheters used for pressure measurements or fluid administration, because of their proximate position to the heart (even though they have a fairly high resistance) can also deliver a lethal shock to the myocardium because of high current density. The shock level required to produce such an effect in humans is on the order of 0.0001 A (0.1 mA or 100 microamps). This current is only one tenth the level required for perceptible discomfort at the level of the skin.

Current Density.—Why does a macroshock of 1 mA at the skin only result in discomfort, whereas a much smaller microshock at the myocardium results in ventricular fibrillation? The current density generated by a 1 mA macroshock delivered to the skin has *insufficient current density at the level of the heart* to cause fibrillation. The much smaller microshock delivered to the heart may have sufficient current density. This principle may be used to beneficial effect if anticipated and applied appropriately. Electrical defibrillation of the heart is based on delivering a critical current density in the cardiac conduction system of the ventricle so as to cause complete, but transient, depolarization of all myocardium. During recovery from the depolarization, a regular cardiac rhythm may resume. A defibrillator is essentially a large capacitor designed to deliver energy through electrodes. External defibrillation—defibrillation through electrode paddles placed on the thorax—requires an energy level of about 25 to 400 J to effect an alteration of heart rhythm. As expected from our discussion of current density, internal defibrillation—defibrillation through electrodes placed on the heart directly—requires an energy level of only a few joules to effect an alteration of heart rhythm.

Pathway of Shock Current

There are two connections that are necessary before current flows in a completed circuit. One is a connection to a source of higher electrical potential, and the other is a connection to a lower source. As unlikely as it seems, there are many possibilities for a human surrounded by electrical apparatus to achieve these conditions. Electrical instruments may be purposely attached to a human, or the human may inadvertently contact an instrument or electrical device.

Purposeful Connection.—Patients or subjects are purposely attached to electrical devices and instruments for both diagnostic and therapeutic purposes. An electrocautery or a pacemaker wire is supposed to deliver a controlled amount of electrical energy to a specific part of the body, but may provide one of the sites of connection that complete an electrical circuit capable of shock. Although one may consider that an electrode or transducer cable carries signal *from* the patient to the instrument, the cable is a potential two-way street that is capable of carrying shock from the instrument's power supply *to* the patient.

Inadvertent Connection.—Patients or subjects also may inadvertently contact both a higher and lower source of electrical potential.

High potential sources may come from a light switch, a motorized bed control, or an instrument case that is casually contacted. Low potential sources may be any ground path. Both are described below. Extreme care of design and manufacture is taken in modern instruments and electrical devices destined for a hospital environment, and special procedures and devices are used to prevent patients from simultaneously contacting sources of high and low electrical potential. These devices and procedures are not panaceas; all afford only limited protection, and may be improperly used or maintained.

Sources of Electrical Potential

The most obvious source of electrical hazard is the high potential lead ("live" or "hot" wire as opposed to the "neutral" or "cold" wire) from a wall outlet or power cord (the cable that runs from the wall outlet to the electrical device or instrument). Covers and containers over the instrument chassis (also called the housing or case), and insulation and coverings over electrical wires and connectors, serve the vital function of protecting the user from direct connection to the power source. An experimental subject or patient could directly contact a hot wire if grossly hazardous conditions were present, such as an exposed electrical cord or wall outlet. In the course of instrument repair or maintenance, because these first-line safety devices are removed to facilitate repair, this type of hazard is much more apparent. However, it is this very covering that may obscure a defect and lead to an inadvertent and indirect contact with a source of electrical potential.

Electrical Connections.—What happens to electrical power wires when they enter the case of an instrument? In general, these insulated live and neutral wires are distributed to the various components within the instrument. They are physically separated and insulated from the case of the instrument by airspace (a very poor conductor) or an insulating material. For good safety practice (mandatory in devices intended for patient connection) the electrical power is *isolated* by a transformer. This device floats the electrical potential so that it is not referenced to ground; we will see shortly why this is an important safety feature. The purpose of this physical insulation and electrical isolation is to prevent a source of voltage potential from coming in contact with the instrument case (which is usually made of metal) and causing the case to serve as a voltage source. If there is improper insulation or isolation, a shock may occur if a source of high potential contacts the case of the instrument, and then a human touches the case and simultaneously *completes the circuit by touching ground* (Fig 1–6).

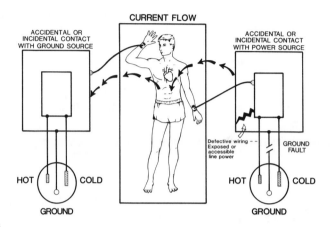

FIG 1–6.

Shock hazard—macroshock. An example of a macroshock caused by high potential and a ground fault. Line power contacts the case of an electrical device or instrument that either has no ground or has a ground fault. The person accidentally touches or, through a device, is incidentally connected to the case of the device which receives full line power. The person completes the circuit by accidentally touching or incidentally is connected to the case of an instrument that is grounded, or any other source of ground. Depending on skin resistance and current pathway through the body, the effects of macroshock may vary from skin pain to burns to death.

Where redundant insulation has been used to prevent the instrument case from serving as a source of high potential, the equipment is labeled "double insulated."

Leakage Current.—In addition to the considerations related to shock caused by line current—current available by direct contact with the power source—there are shock considerations related to *leakage current,* which is the small current caused by indirect contact with the power source. With respect to the power source, the instrument case has finite resistance (usually very large) and finite capacitance (usually very small). All power lines, motors, electrical equipment, and instruments generate an electrical field (which may be observed as "noise" while recording the desired signal) during their operation. These electrical fields can actually generate a voltage on the case of the instrument in which they are contained or on a nearby instrument through the resistance and capacitance of the case—the *resistive and capacitive coupling* effect. Again, current will flow through an object (like a human) which contacts the case and simultaneously *completes the circuit by contacting ground* (Fig 1–7). Leakage currents may be on the order of a

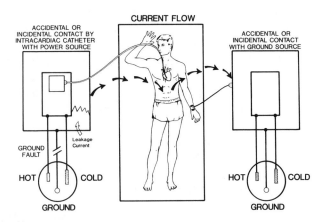

FIG 1–7.
Shock hazard—microshock. An example of a microshock caused by a leakage current. A small potential occurs on the case of an electrical device or instrument through capacitive coupling. As described in Figure 1–6, the person simultaneously contacts the source of potential and a ground source. However, this time the pathway of current through the body is a low-resistance intracardiac catheter. Even though shock current is small, a critical current density is achieved in the heart that results in ventricular fibrillation.

few milliamps, and definitely pose a shock hazard if skin resistance is reduced or if a cardiac catheter is in place.

Instrument manufacturers and clinical engineering departments spend the greatest amount of care and attention in eliminating or minimizing the effects of capacitive coupling and other small sources of leakage currents that find their way to the case of the instrument. However, none of these methods of insulation or isolation is foolproof for the purposes of either preventing shock or reducing noise during signal measurement. Therefore, it is almost universal that a third connecting wire has been added to the electrical cord called the "ground" wire.

Grounding

The object of the ground wire is to provide an alternative and preferred pathway for voltage potential and leakage current, which is present on the case of an instrument, to find its way to ground other than through a human.

Ground Wire.—The ground wire is physically connected to the case of the instrument, usually on the inside. It joins the insulated hot and neutral wires within the power cord and terminates in the round spike of the typical 110 VAC power plug. However, *unlike* those parts of the wall receptacle that carry the hot and neutral potentials back to the power generating station, this ground part of the receptacle terminates a relatively short distance away within the building structure onto a large conductor called a bus, which is literally connected to ground. That is, it physically joins a metal spike that is driven substantially into the earth. This bus, the ground wires connected to the bus, and the instrument cases that are connected to the ground wires are at "ground" or zero potential. Therefore, should the case be contacted by a source of potential that is referenced to ground, such as either the hot or neutral wires of the electrical source or the resistive or capacitive coupling of the electromagnetic field, current flow will be diverted to ground because of the very low resistance pathway of the ground system. Therefore, no large potential difference will develop on the case.

Older equipment may not have a ground connection (it will *not* be allowed in a hospital environment) and may be made safer by replacing the existing power cord with a grounded (three-wire) power cord and by connecting the ground wire to an appropriate place on the instrument case.

Limitations of Grounding.—Improper grounding may, itself, pose a shock hazard. Potential differences, and therefore the capability of current flow, can exist between the cases of two instruments *each of which is incapable of delivering a shock by itself, and each of which is grounded.* This occurs because all ground wires and buses have a small but finite resistance and, when there is current flow, there is some generation of electrical potential (Ohm's law).

Usually, a cord with a grounding wire of substantial length is connected to an outlet with a long run of wire that connects to the building's ground bus and finally reaches earth (and therefore true grounding). When more than one instrument is attached to a patient or subject, and if there is current flow from the case of one instrument through its ground, or if a remote device on the same ground bus as these two instruments is discharging a large current flow into the bus, then the actual ground conditions at the case of each instrument may be slightly different. That is, a potential difference can exist between the two instrument grounds and therefore between two case grounds, or between any case ground and any other source of ground the patient might be touched by or might be connected to. As a result a small potential difference may develop. This could, for example, be sufficient to result in a shock hazard if connected to a pathway of low resistance into the heart, such as an intracardiac catheter.

Testing for Ground Function.—The instrument user can check for a gross malfunction of the operation of the ground system, *but not for its appropriate function*. Use a VOM to check the resistance between the instrument case and the hot, neutral, and ground spike of the instrument plug. There should be a very large resistance (an "open" circuit) between the case and the hot or neutral blades of the plug, and no resistance (continuity) between the case and the ground spike. Then check the wall receptacle. A voltmeter should show full potential (e.g., 110 VAC) between the hot and neutral slots and between the hot and ground slot. No voltage potential indicates either that the circuit is not energized or that there is a fault in the ground or neutral wire. However, the user should be warned that electrical codes specify the types and quantities of values from the above tests which are beyond the capabilities of the VOM to measure accurately and which require special test instruments.

Other Electrical Safety and Warning Devices
There are a few other safety devices that should be mentioned.

The Electrical Power Plug.—The three-pronged plug (hot, neutral, and ground) also ensures that the hot and neutral wires of the plug are mated to the AC wall outlet in the proper configuration. Inspection of a new wall outlet shows that the two slotted connections of the outlet are of unequal size: the larger slot is connected to the neutral wire (white wire) and accommodates the blade of the neutral wire of the instrument plug, and the smaller slot is connected to the hot wire (black or deep-color wire) and contacts the blade of the hot wire of the instrument plug.

Until recently, the proper sequence of mating of the blades of the plug to outlet was important, because the switch that controlled power to the instrument was single pole. That is, it only controlled a single wire—the hot wire—as it entered the case. If the wall outlet were mis-wired, if the grounding spike of the plug were torn off and the plug reversed in its socket, or if the plug had two equal-sized blades that allowed insertion in the wall socket in either direction, grave consequences were possible. First, the instrument was potentially energized all the time because the source of high potential was coming in on the unswitched side of the circuit. Although current could only flow if the device contacted a path of low potential, this ground path could be through a person who managed to contact some energized part of the device and simultaneously completed the circuit by touching ground. Worse, in some older instruments, the neutral wire was also connected to the case to act as a chassis ground and the reversal of the plug applied the full line potential to the case. This should no longer be possible in a hospital environment. All switches should be double pole—that is, control both hot and neutral wires. Also, the neutral wire should not be connected to case or ground. Additionally, the use of isolated power, such as by a transformer, leaves the power supply floating—that is, the high potential of the transformer is referenced only to the low potential of the transformer, and not to ground. Even if such a voltage potential finds its way to the case, no current will flow between the case and ground.

Ground Fault Detectors.—Another safety device is the ground-fault-circuit-interruptor (GFCI), which is a special type of circuit breaker. This device is built into the wall outlet, or sometimes placed back at the circuit breaker box to monitor a number of wall outlets simultaneously. Normally, there should be equal current flow through the hot and the neutral wires. The GFCI monitors the equality of the current flow. If an imbalance is detected, it is assumed that a ground fault has occurred; that some of the current has found its way from one arm of the circuit to a ground. The GFCI will trip and act as an open switch within the outlet to prevent current flow from either the hot or neutral wires. Another device, the ground fault indicator (GFI) uses the same principle as the GFCI, but its only action is to indicate a fault through a warning light. The typical specification to trip a GFCI or GFI is an imbalance of a few milliamps. If the GFCI trips, do not reset it and do not reoperate the instrument without a careful instrument safety check.

Fuse and Circuit Breakers.—The final safety device is the fuse or circuit breaker that controls the wall outlet or the instrument. *They confer no protection from electrical shock hazard.* At the outset, it must be appreciated that these devices have to be tolerant enough to allow large current flow to avoid the interruption of the operation of the device or the instrument. Therefore, their utility is entirely to protect the wiring within the structure of the building or of the instrument from a large current overload and possible fire. Of course, this is a very important function. A typical fuse or circuit breaker will control a few wall outlets and will be rated at 15 or 20 amps. This will not confer any human protection. Fuses or circuit breakers will be built into most instruments. Here again their rating must be large enough to accommodate the current flow of the instrument, and there is no protection against electrical shock.

Other Safety Hazards

The diversity of instrumentation and their complex modes of operation offer a Pandora's box of safety hazards. Although it is not possible to offer a comprehensive listing of safety hazards, we can review some types of hazards.

Fire and Explosion Hazards

The flow of current through a resistance generates heat, and electrical circuits always pose a fire hazard in addition to a shock hazard. The principles of electrical device design are intended to limit heat production, to dissipate heat content to avoid a large rise of temperature, to use nonflammable materials, and to provide current limiting devices such as fuses. Fire safety continues to occupy attention and requires fastidious attention to detail.

Hazardous and flammable compounds cannot be introduced into areas in which human subjects are present. Flammable anesthetics have been irrevocably banned from all operating rooms.

Mechanical Hazards

These fall into two categories: instruments that have moving parts, and the more gross possibility that a piece of an instrument or the bulk of an instrument collides with a person. Moving parts include pens on recorders, tables with cradles that turn, or instrument parts that are meant to be in close proximity and move around a patient, such as the detecting head of a scintillation camera. Careful inspection and observation of mode of operation are necessary in operating these devices.

The more gross type of mechanical hazard occurs when something not tied down falls on the subject, or the subject collides with the object. The law of gravity is premier—only permanently mounted objects should be allowed above a patient. The tops of instruments should not be used as storage platforms for any other nonsecured equipment, or for hazardous materials such as tools, chemicals, or cleaning solvents. All devices, equipment, and material not germane to the study at hand should be removed from the area while the subject is present. Maintenance of equipment and floors in a clean and dry state is mandatory.

Hazards Peculiar to the Instrument or to the Experimental Design

These flaws and potential problems should come to light in the course of experimental design and shakeout. All instruments will eventually fail to perform properly, and their mode of failure should be of particular concern to the investigators. For example, electrode cables and electrolyte skin patches will frequently fail in use and no signal will be present at that time. This may be a nuisance and interrupt the data collection, or it could seriously impair the ability to make a time-dependent decision. Machines that act on signal and deliver substances back to the patient may have catastrophic failure modes with drug delivery markedly over or under the intended amount. The final opportunity to detect and prevent these problems usually comes at the time of instrument calibration (chapter 9). This is another reason to perform this calibration immediately before its use, and to take frequent calibrations during the course of the experiment to verify proper operation. Routine maintenance checks and preventative maintenance may also reduce these failures (chapter 10).

Safety Regulations

Multiple agencies are concerned with safety policy. Local institutional policies are further bolstered by municipal and state codes, by insurance carriers, and by the Joint Commission on the Accreditation of Hospitals (JCAH).

Published Standards for Instrument Safety

Underwriters Laboratories (U.L.) is an independent, not-for-profit organization testing for public safety. U.L. develops safety specifications and inspects and certifies that samples of instruments submitted to U.L. meet certain of their published specifications. Many institutions will require that all equipment have the U.L. certifications relevant to hospital safety. When equipment does not have U.L. certification, a hospital, insurance carrier, or municipal or state code may demand that it be tested and meet certain standards before use is permitted. Sometimes it is possible to retrofit or alter equipment to meet those standards. However, the time and expense needed to test and modify instruments to meet stringent safety specifications make this difficult. Instrument buyers should continue to insist that manufacturers of medical equipment meet published standards and submit such equipment for certification before marketing.

U.L. 544.—One example of an accepted standard for instruments is the *Standard for Safety: Medical and Dental Equipment (U.L. 544).** Although this document is most commonly cited for its electrical safety

*Underwriters Laboratories, Inc., Publications Stock, 333 Pfingston Rd., Northbrook, IL 60062.

standards, it is actually a comprehensive document that covers all manner of electrical and mechanical construction and operation of medical and dental equipment. This document is widely recognized and accepted as a safety standard for medical equipment by agencies that certify hospitals, by insurance carriers, and by municipal codes. There are other equally stringent and comprehensive standards that are accepted.

2

Properties of Biologic Signals

The process of measurement starts with a knowledge of what signal is to be measured and what properties characterize the signal. This is not as obvious as it seems. It may be possible to measure the behavior of a biologic organism by one or more signals that are part of that organism's behavior (some of which may not even be known), and the observer will have to decide which signal to measure. For example, to characterize the behavior of cardiac activity, it is possible to measure bioelectricity, pressure, flow, motion, and biochemistry. Cardiac activity was incompletely characterized until the end of the 19th century because it was not recognized to include bioelectricity along with previously described pressure and flow generation. The decision and the technology to measure one aspect of biologic behavior in preference to another is important. Wiggers commented that the entire course of cardiovascular physiology would have changed had flow been easy to measure and pressure difficult. The appropriate application of instrumentation requires that a few questions be answered about the characteristics of the biologic signal under study.

WHAT YOU NEED TO KNOW

1. The correct application of instrumentation for signal measurement requires a priori knowledge about the characteristics of that signal, including its physical form, location, and time base.

2. A special example of the time base characteristics of a signal is its periodicity. Periodic signals, signals that appear to be repeated over a constant period of time, are important practically because they allow multiple opportunities for observation.

3. Periodic signals are also important conceptually because they can be described by their frequency content or bandwidth. One of the characteristics common to both signals and instruments is their bandwidth.

4. The frequency spectrum of a signal can be obtained by direct knowledge of the characteristics of the signal, by consulting a data base of information about the signal, or by formal analysis. As a first approximation, a visual analysis of the signal is useful.

Signal Characteristics

Definition: *A biologic signal is a detectable piece of information that characterizes some or all of the behavior (usually the structure or function) of the tissue or biologic process under study.*

Before a signal can be measured successfully by an instrument, it is necessary to know or to derive some characteristics about its form, location, time base, and frequency content. This is because instruments have limitations of the signal characteristics that they can observe by both design and physical properties (see chapters 4 through 9), and it is necessary to match the properties of the instrumentation with those of the biologic signal. Sometimes, a new study or investigation will be built on an older one, and this information on signal characteristics is already available to guide the study. Frequently, the information is not available or is incomplete. Then, pilot studies will have to be performed and, initially, inference will have to be used about these signal characteristics during measurement. This initial study or inference should give way to further refinement in the process of measurement as more of the signal characteristics are determined.

Signal Form
There are only two forms of matter, including biologic signals: mass and energy. These two basic forms can be expressed as subtypes, described below.

Bioelectricity.—The origin of bioelectrical signals is ionic, and therefore these are a special type of biochemical signal. While a transmembrane potential exists in almost all cells, spontaneous or provocable (caused by the application of a stimulus) sudden change of electrical potential is present in intact and individual cells (action potential) of the brain (electroencephalogram) and nerve tissue, the heart (electrocardiogram), and striated and smooth muscle (electromyogram) and in specialized organs of certain animals.

Radiation.—Radiation is characterized as either ionizing or nonionizing. Spontaneous (generated by a normal process of the organism) biologic radiation is always nonionizing, as in the case of heat, sound, and light. Heat production and heat content (temperature) are present as the byproduct of almost all chemical reactions and physical processes. Rarely, light is emitted by special purpose organs of some primitive creatures. Sound is generated by motion of part or all of the organism under study and by the flow of fluids within an organism.

Induced (caused by the observer) radiation can either be ionizing or nonionizing. Because nonionizing radiation has proven to be very safe, it is especially valuable in studies of fragile tissues (like humans) and during repetitive studies. Light is an example of electromagnetic nonionizing radiation that is sometimes used for studies. Ultrasound and Doppler ultrasound are examples of acoustic nonionizing radiation used for study of structure and physiologic function, whereas magnetic resonance imaging is an example of electromagnetic nonionizing radiation used for study of structure and chemical processes.

Ionizing radiation is further characterized as emission and transmission. The primary example of transmitted radiation is the x-ray, which is used for study of structure and physiologic function. Examples of emission radiation are the rays and particles from the decay of radionuclide tracers which have similar uses to transmitted radiation, but are also widely used in biochemical measurements.

Chemical.—All biologic processes involve chemical reactions. The monitoring of such reactions and their end-products is frequently of interest.

Mass.—A basic property of all organisms is their mass. It is sometimes desirable to monitor the mass output of some biologic process. An example might be the amount of product from a chemical reaction.

Flow.—Fluid transfer within a system is a special example of mass transfer as a signal that may be of interest to measure, such as blood flow in the heart or vascular tree or air flow in the bronchial tree.

Pressure.—Enclosed spaces within animals are frequently pressurized, and the operating characteristics or evidence of malfunction of that system can be determined in part by measurement of pressure. Examples are pressures in various blood vessels to characterize various parts of the vascular tree; pressure in the pleural space to characterize the operating parameters of the lungs; and pressure in the cranial vault to determine abnormal space occupying lesions.

Motion.—Movement of an animal is frequently characteristic of the behavior of an animal. Translational motion is seen in locomotion of the body. Translation and rotation are frequently seen in complex motion activities, such as cardiac contraction and lung inflation.

Location of Signal
The locus of the signal is an important determinant in the application of instrumentation. For example, although electrocardiographic signals can be detected anywhere on the surface of the skin of an animal with a heart, the signal may be better detected or may contain some additional information at some specific sites. If we take this example a step further, some specific aspects of cardiac electrophysiology can be determined only by the application of intracardiac electrocardiography or the application of electrodes to specific sites within the myocardium or myocardial cell. It may not be immediately recognized that one site or location confers better or different information than another site. For example, detection of arterial pressure could be performed in any artery large enough to admit a catheter. But, in some forms of analysis, it may be very useful to measure pressure at the aortic root. For many signals, the amplitude diminishes as one moves away from the site of signal generation, and the possibility of including noise or error increases.

The Time Base Characteristics of the Signal
There are a few questions to be answered about the time characteristics of the signal under study. How often does the signal occur, and is it a spontaneous event or a provoked event under experimental control? What is the duration of the signal? Is the signal periodic?

Rate, Spontaneity, and Duration of a Signal.—Events that occur uncommonly or not spontaneously require special vigilance in the application of instrumentation. A rarely occurring cardiac arrhythmic event may require many hours of the application of instrumentation, data gathering, and analysis before it is detected. The possibility that an infrequent spontaneous event may go undetected is high because the observer cannot afford the time or effort to gather such data, because the organism may not tolerate the prolonged application of instrumentation and because the reliability of instruments sometimes declines in proportion to the duration of application (although the rate of this deterioration may be minimized).

In the detection of such a signal, many experimenters have opted for systems in which they can evoke or provoke the signal rather than awaiting its spontaneous occurrence. For example, stimulation of cardiac arrhythmias may be substituted for spontaneous events: the assumptions of such an experiment are many, and include that the evoked and the spontaneous event have the same physiologic basis and clinical significance.

Short-lived events, especially when they are of low amplitude and high frequency content, complicate the application of instrumentation.

Periodicity

A special example of the time-based characteristics of signals is their period. Signals are either periodic or nonperiodic. When a signal—even one that has a complex form or shape—repeats itself exactly after a time, it is called periodic. Examples of biologic signals that closely (although sometimes not exactly) fit the definition of periodic behavior are many spontaneous and stimulated electrophysiologic, cardiac, and respiratory signals.

Periodic signals are especially important for two reasons. First, they offer an opportunity for repetitive observation and therefore increase the chance of the detection of an event; and, when observations are averaged, periodic signals enhance the confidence in the information that can be gathered about such an event (see chapter 3, "Random Error"). Second, periodic signals fuse one of the important concepts of biologic characteristics of a signal, which is the province of this chapter, with one of the performance characteristics of instruments, which is the province of the next few chapters. That characteristic is frequency content or bandwidth, which we will define shortly.

Periodic Waves—The Sine Wave

It is especially convenient to describe signals in a graphical form or waveform. In order to do this, let me briefly jog the reader's memory of high school geometry. There are a few things one needs to describe the simplest of periodic waves—the sinusoidal (sine or cosine) wave.

They are the frequency (or period), the amplitude (height or level) and, when describing more than one sinusoidal wave, the phase relationship (or relative angle) between the waves.

Period and Frequency.—One needs to know how often the wave is repeating itself or "beating." This is called its *frequency*, which is given in cycles per unit time. When the unit of time is a second, the frequency can be expressed in Hertz (Hz) or cycles per second (cps). Alternately, it's just fine to describe the *period* of the wave, which is the time or duration it takes for a sine wave to complete one cycle. Frequency and period are simply calculated as the inverse of each other: a frequency of 1 Hz would have a duration of 1 sec; a frequency of 2 Hz would have a duration of 0.5 sec.

There is a simple relationship between sine waves that occur at different frequencies. A sine wave of 10 Hz (or a period of 0.1 sec) beats or cycles ten times more often than a wave of 1 Hz. Because it is a recurrent theme with respect to electrical power and electrical interference, we repeat that municipal electrical supplies (AC electrical power) in the United States are generated at 50 to 60 Hz.

Amplitude.—One needs to know how tall the wave is. This is called the *amplitude,* which has the dimensions of whatever quantity is being measured. The amplitude of a sine wave changes over time. However, the relationship between any point on a sine wave and its peak and trough are entirely predictable because the form or shape of a sine wave can be described by an exact mathematical formula.* Frequently, the term *amplitude* is reserved to describe the height or level of the peak of the wave. Because a sinusoidal wave is symmetrical, the height of the peak about the midpoint of the wave is the same as, but in opposite direction to, the valley of the wave.

Sometimes, as in discussions of electrical power, the root mean square (RMS) of a sinusoidal wave is used to describe a type of amplitude of the wave. The peak amplitude of a sinusoidal wave is equal to the RMS amplitude multiplied by the square root of 2. Therefore, when the amplitude of a sine wave is discussed, the reader will have to pay attention to (or question) whether a particular amplitude, or peak or RMS amplitude is used, because the difference can be considerable.

*The formula that describes the shape of a sine wave is as follows:

$$x(t) = A \cdot \sin 2 \cdot Pi \cdot f \cdot t$$

where x is the amplitude of a sine wave that has a peak amplitude A, a frequency f, at any time, t.

Typically, electrical voltage at the wall outlet in the United States is a simple sinusoid which has an amplitude of about 115 VAC RMS. The amplitude of the voltage varies between (about) $+163$ and -163 VAC.

Phase.—Finally, when more than one sinusoidal wave is described, one needs to know the timing relationship between the waves. This is done by comparing a known point on one wave (like the midpoint or peak) to the comparable point on the other wave and measuring the timing relationship between them. This could be expressed in units of time. However, because a wave repeats itself every 360° (or every 2 Pi radians), it is common to express this timing relationship as the *angle or phase* relationship between the waves expressed in units of degrees or radians, rather than in units of time.

Unbeknown to most users, municipal power supplies in the United States are generated as three sinusoids (so-called three-phase power) at 60 Hz. Each sine wave is identical in frequency and amplitude but is offset in phase by 120°, or ⅔ Pi radians.

Periodic Behavior of Simple Signals

There are a large number of examples from everyday life that qualify as periodic events, and that might be described by the use of the same concepts that describe sine waves.

Rotation of the Earth.—Perhaps the most common example of periodic behavior is the motion of the earth due to its daily cycle of rotation. This may be described in terms of the motion of a point on the surface of the earth in relationship to the sun. Imagine sitting in an equatorial paradise, reading this chapter, sipping a cool drink (the above not supplied with book purchase), and measuring the distance from your location to the sun (Fig 2–1). As the earth rotates with a period of one day (a frequency of 1/day or 1/86,400 Hz) the amplitude of your spot on earth slightly increases and slightly decreases with respect to the distance from the sun. Now, although the average amplitude of this distance is 93 million miles, we are actually more affected by the peak amplitude changes of only about 8,000 miles that occur daily. The graph of the motion of a location on the earth as a distance from the sun plotted over time is a simple sine wave. The rotational motion of many celestial bodies at their equator is almost a simple sine wave and periodic—only the prophet Joshua could make this motion aperiodic by requesting that the sun and the moon stand still.*

*Joshua 10:12–13.

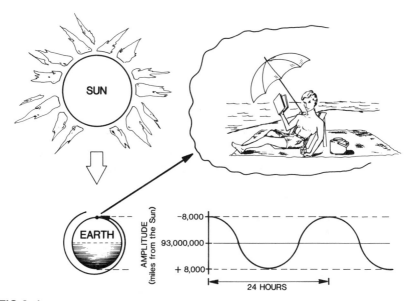

FIG 2–1.
Simple periodic motion of the earth. The rotation of the earth is an example of simple harmonic (sine wave) motion. While the average amplitude of the distance from the earth to the sun is 93 million miles, the diurnal variation of 8,000 miles has a much more immediate impact on our lives.

Pure Tones.—Sound waves have frequency and amplitude that can be sensed by the ear. What we call pitch is our sensory perception of the frequency of sound waves, and what we call loudness is our sensory perception of amplitude of sound waves. Given the variations and subtleties of music (further discussed below) it seems difficult to express those sound waves only in such simple terms. Yet, at its most basic level, music is a synthesis of multiple simple sine waves of different frequency and amplitude.

The most simple musical sounds or tones are described by a single frequency. An "A" above middle "C" has a frequency of 440 Hz*, whereas a middle "C" has a frequency of about 261.63 Hz. Notes repeat themselves at frequency intervals of an octave, which is a doubling or a halving of the frequency. For example, we will have occasion to return to the great octave "C" which is two octaves below middle "C"; it has a frequency of 65.41 Hz. Our ears are sensitive devices for

*The London convention of 1939 defined the chromatic musical scale of 12 notes based on the frequency of this "A." All other notes then have a precise mathematical relationship to this frequency.

discriminating among these frequencies; however, like instruments, we do have limitations. The range of frequencies that our ears can hear is from about 20 to 20,000 Hz.

Because music is such a useful analogy to biologic signals, and because component stereo systems are an everyday analogy of biomedical instruments, we will have occasion to return to both in later sections of the book.

Periodic Behavior of Slightly More Complex Signals

There are some signals that can be characterized by waveforms that are almost sinusoids. The curve of their waveform deviates from a sine wave, in that the amplitude over the period does not exactly follow that of a sine wave, and its form and period may vary a bit from cycle to cycle. Nevertheless, some aspects of a simple sine wavelike analysis of frequency and amplitude are appropriate.

Windshield Wipers.—There is a monotony and certainty—which is reassuring while you're driving in a rainstorm—to the motion of windshield wipers. Imagine sitting in the driver's seat of a car and observing the motion of the wiper that is directly in front of your eyes (Fig 2–2). It swings from a horizontal position on your right up to a vertical position on your left, then back to horizontal again. Because of the way that the wipers and their supporting devices are constructed, you can't really change the amount of motion (amplitude) that the wipers go through, only the rate of the cycle (frequency).

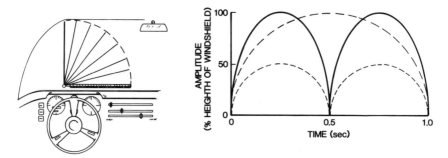

Fig 2–2.
Periodic motion of windshield wipers. A common example of a periodic signal from everyday life is the motion of windshield wipers. The tip of the wiper blade moves from the bottom of the windshield to the top, then back again. The period (or its inverse, frequency) can be varied by the driver. Different points on the wiper can be seen to move different vertical distances. Although the motion is periodic, the shape is not exactly that of a sine wave.

On many cars, you can adjust the rate of cycling and get the blades to cycle a single time, perhaps to clear the windshield of some rain or debris. The motion of the wiper won't repeat itself until you make it do so—it's a one-shot deal, or nonperiodic motion. Additional adjustments of rate control keep the wipers cycling back and forth, or periodically. Some cars have a switch that allows a varied gradation—from very slow up to fast—of the speed of the wipers. In my car, the slow, medium, and fast periods are 5 sec, 1 sec, and 0.5 sec, respectively. That would correspond to 12 cycles/min (0.2 Hz), 60 cycles/min (1 Hz), and 120 cycles/min (2 Hz), respectively.

Now consider the motion of a point on the wiper blade—say the end. From the inside of the car, you see it move from about the middle of the windshield up to near the upper left corner of the windshield. In terms of the height of the windshield, it's moving from the bottom to nearly the top and then back again to the bottom. We measure this amplitude in inches or centimeters. The maximum distance from the top to the bottom of my windshield is about 20 in, or 50 cm.

Not all parts of the wiper move the same amplitude up and down on the windshield. Think about a point perhaps halfway along the wiper. It starts at the bottom of the windshield, but during the cycle it only makes it about halfway up the windshield before falling back again—a moderate amplitude motion. Furthermore, in terms of this up/down motion or amplitude, there's the part near the center of the wiper blade that hardly makes it at all up and down on the windshield—a low-amplitude motion. Wipers on other vehicles may be longer or shorter than mine. The up/down motion and therefore the amplitude of the tip of a wiper on a municipal bus is much larger than my car, while the end point of the wiper blade of some of those spiffy sports cars has considerably less amplitude (small consolation to me).

The major similarity between this motion and the examples of simple sinusoidal motion is that very important features, such as frequency and amplitude, can be used to describe both. The major difference is that the variation of amplitude over the period of motion of the windshield wiper is not exactly the same as a sine wave.

Circadian Rhythms.—When the period of a biologic rhythm is a day (frequency of 1/day) the rhythm is referred to as *circadian* or *diurnal*. Core temperature—the temperature of the bulk of the central body tissues such as the heart, the brain, and the blood circulating through them—shows a circadian rhythm. With some exceptions, such as a fever or the ovulatory cycle, the daily temperature cycle shows the lowest temperature or amplitude in the early morning hours, increases throughout the day until the early evening, then slowly decreases throughout the night and reaches a minimum amplitude before arising.

Diurnal variations are seen in other organ systems. Serum cortisol levels have daily repetitive swings of amplitude: highest in the morning and lowest in the evening. Wake/sleep cycles are diurnal, except perhaps when interrupted under special circumstances. Even blood pressure swings in most people throughout a daily cycle: lowest in amplitude in the early morning hours except for a rapid and moderate increase in amplitude before arising, and then slowly increasing throughout the day before a maximum amplitude in the afternoon, then decreasing through the evening and late night.

More Complex Periodic Signals

There is a set of even more complex signals that really doesn't look like sine waves. Their major claim to similarity is that they have a reasonably consistent frequency and amplitude over repetitive periods of the signal—something we can probably call periodic. However, it's not so obvious how to fully characterize these signals.

Respiratory System.—Many respiratory events involving the mechanical aspects of ventilation are reasonably periodic. Their frequency and their amplitude over the period of the signal are more or less consistent. The basic period is the duration of a respiratory cycle (usually expressed in seconds or milliseconds) or its frequency is the respiratory rate (usually expressed in dimensions of min^{-1}). The signals, which more or less are consistent with the definition of periodic signals, include pressure and flow into and out of the lungs (Fig 2–3), motion of the chest wall, and tension development and shortening of the dia-

FIG 2–3.
Periodic respiratory signal. The expiratory flow rate of a human is a close approximation of a periodic signal. Over a few respiratory cycles, the period and shape of the waveform are reasonably consistent. Here is the expiratory flow signal of a human during light exercise. The frequency is 0.42 Hz, which is more commonly expressed as 25 breaths per minute. The minimum flow velocity is 0 L/sec, whereas the maximum is about 1 L/sec.

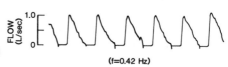

FLOW (L/sec) 1.0 · 0

(f=0.42 Hz)

phragm and respiratory muscles. However, the shape of these wave-forms is somewhat different from the shape of a sine wave.

Cardiovascular Behavior.—Many cardiovascular events involving both the electrical and the mechanical aspects of the heart and circulation are reasonably periodic in that their frequency and their amplitude during the period are more or less consistent. The basic cardiovascular period is the duration of the heartbeat (usually expressed in sec or msec) or its frequency is the heart rate (usually expressed in b/min or Hz). Electrical depolarization of the ventricle, shortening of cardiac muscle, and the pulsing nature of the blood pressure all occur at the frequency of the heart rate. The units used to describe each of these events and the amplitudes of these events are different. The shape and the nuance of each of these events are also different. The shape of an ECG looks vastly different from that of the shortening of the left ventricle, which in turn looks vastly different than the waveform of the arterial or pulmonary artery blood pressures (Fig 2–4).

Music.—Let's return to our earlier example of musical tones. What is the difference between the pure tone of a great octave "C"—say one produced by a tuning fork—and the "C" produced by a piano or clarinet? In all instruments, this "C" is defined as a frequency of about 65.41 Hz; but the difference between instruments is the variation of the waveform over this basic or fundamental frequency. Each instrument produces its own complex and subtle variation of amplitude during the basic or defined frequency of that note or sound. The shape of the waveform of a piano is distinctly different from that of a clarinet, yet each waveform of a great octave "C" repeats itself 65.41 times per second.

These subtle variations are produced by including additional higher frequencies within the waveform of the basic frequency. The great octave "C" of a musical instrument includes not only the basic tone frequency of 65.41 Hz, which is called the *fundamental* or *first harmonic* of the sound, but also includes frequencies that are integer multiples of the fundamental—2 times 65.41 Hz, 3 times 65.41 Hz, etc. These are called the *additional harmonics* of the fundamental, or the *overtones*. The graphical representation of the note from a clarinet gives us a good opportunity to concretize the relationship between complex and simple (sinusoidal) waveforms (Fig 2–5). In part, the "C" note is sinusoidal because it has a predictable fundamental frequency (the wave repeats itself at a known frequency or period) and predictable variation

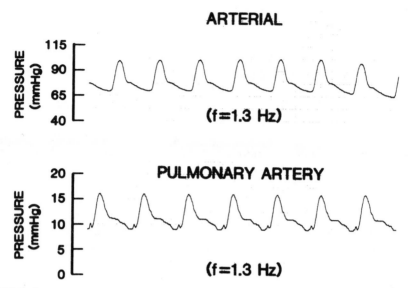

FIG 2–4.
Periodic cardiovascular pressure signals. Many cardiovascular events are close approximations of a periodic signal, because period and waveform are usually consistent for a few
heartbeats. Here are the arterial *(top)* and pulmonary artery *(bottom)* pressure signals from
a human measured in the supine position while at rest. The frequency of both signals is
1.3 Hz, which is more commonly expressed as 78 beats per minute. The minimum arterial
pressure is about 65 mm Hg, whereas the maximum is about 105 mm Hg. The minimum
pulmonary artery pressure is about 9 mm Hg, whereas the maximum is about 16 mm Hg.

FIG 2–5.
Example of a complex periodic
waveform—the great octave "C" note
of a clarinet. The waveform is
considered periodic because, despite
the complexity of its shape, it repeats
itself at a constant frequency. Here the
frequency is 65 Hz.

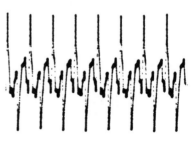

of amplitude over that frequency (the amplitudes of successive notes can be exactly superimposed over the period of the note). In part, the "C" note is different from a sinusoid because its variation of amplitude is more complex, and appears to include additional sinusoidal waves within the basic waveform.

This concept of the composition of a complex but periodic waveform—a series that consists of a basic sine wave and additional sine waves—is based on one of the important mathematical theorems that governs the relationship between the characteristics of signals and the performance of instruments.

Frequency Content or Bandwidth

Having just run through a series of examples of simple and more complex waveforms, the reader should have been left with the impression that there is something unique about periodic waveforms. But is there a principle that emerges from all this? Yes. From this we learn that *it is always possible to decompose a complex periodic signal into a series of simple sine waves*. This principle is based on the Fourier (pronounced *For-ee-ay*) theorem. From this we define the frequency content or bandwidth of a waveform or signal as *the range of frequencies of simple sinusoidal waves that compose the waveform of the signal*.

Why Analyze a Complex Periodic Signal?

We would like to know the frequency content or bandwidth that composes a periodic waveform in order to select an instrument that has an appropriate frequency response. Ideally, this frequency response of the instrument would fully cover the range of the frequency content of the signal. One of the major characteristics and limitations of the function of instruments is their frequency response or bandwidth. At places throughout the book, we will point out the errors that occur in the measurement of signals when the bandwidth of the instrument is less than that of the signal.

The Fourier (Spectral) Analysis

Although it's fairly easy to see how to synthesize or add together a complex waveform from simple sine waves, it is not so obvious how to analyze a complex waveform so as to discern of what simple sine waves it is made. In fact, theoretically a complex waveform might require an infinite series of simple sinusoidal waves of different frequencies, amplitudes, and phase relationship. The analysis of a periodic waveform by use of the Fourier Theorem is called a *spectral* or *Fourier analysis*. It contains the information used to determine the bandwidth or the frequency content of the signal.

The Zero Frequency Term (The Average).—The information contained in the spectral analysis consists, as expected, of sinusoidal waves of different frequencies, amplitude, and phase. The first frequency is the zero "frequency" term. By analogy to electrical power, it is also called the DC term. This also is identical to what we call the arithmetic average of the signal. In the spectral analysis, this term and all subsequent terms are measured as an amplitude that has dimensions of the same units as that of the signal (e.g., mV, mm Hg, L/min, etc.).

This zero frequency term is usually an important value. In fact, sometimes this zero frequency term, DC or average, is the only part of the spectral analysis of interest. When we talk about the average temperature during a day, the average rainfall in a year, a baseball player's batting average over a season, or the mean arterial pressure during a heartbeat, we are ignoring the variations of each of these during the period in favor of a simple and useful piece of information.

Sometimes, the zero frequency term or average is not so important to the description of a signal. This can occur because of mathematical or conceptual reasons. Mathematically, the DC or zero frequency term of the spectral analysis becomes unimportant when its amplitude is zero. That doesn't imply that the whole signal is zero, just its average. For example, AC electrical voltage and current at a wall outlet have a mathematical average, or zero frequency (DC) term in the spectral analysis, of zero. (To get across the point that AC electrical energy was not a total bust, it was necessary to invent an "effective" average that is called the RMS level.)

Sometimes, the DC term is unimportant because conceptually the activity and significance of the signal is contained in its variations. For example, on a day-to-night basis we place more importance on the 8,000-mile variation of the amplitude of the earth's distance from the sun than on its average distance of 93 million miles from the sun. That's myopic in the larger scheme of geological and biologic evolution, but appropriate to our daily existence.

The Fundamental Frequency Term (First Harmonic).—The next term in the spectral analysis is the fundamental frequency term. This term begins the series of sinusoids that characterize the variations of the signal. The fundamental is a sinusoid that has a frequency equal to the basic, minimum, or lowest frequency (or 1/period) of the signal. For example, if the basic frequency of the waveform is ½, 2, or 64 Hz, then a first harmonic will be present at ½, 2, or 64 Hz, respectively.

This fundamental frequency or first harmonic will have an amplitude in dimensions of that of the signal (e.g., mV, mm Hg, L/min, etc.), and a phase angle. The phase is used to place this term in the proper timing relationship to subsequent terms. The simplest example of the spectral analysis of a periodic wave is a sine wave itself. The accompanying diagram (Fig 2–6) shows the spectral analysis of the rotation of the earth to which we referred previously. Only two terms are needed to describe the periodic motion of the earth's daily rotation: the zero frequency term with a value of 93 million miles, and the first harmonic term with a value of 8,000 miles. Now we have converted a signal whose graph required a time axis to one whose graph is described entirely in frequency terms. That is, we have gone from the "time domain" to the "frequency domain."

Additional Terms (Second and Higher Harmonics).—Additional terms in the Fourier analysis are present at each integer multiple of the fundamental frequency (e.g., 2, 3, 4, etc.). Analogous to the terms used to describe musical notes, they are called the harmonics of the fundamental. Each term has an amplitude that has the same dimensions as that of the signal (e.g., mV, mm Hg, L/min, etc.) and a phase. However, for purposes of comparison among similar signals, sometimes the amplitude of the first harmonic is used as a reference value against which the amplitude of these higher harmonics is compared. In that case, the amplitude of the first harmonic is used as a denomi-

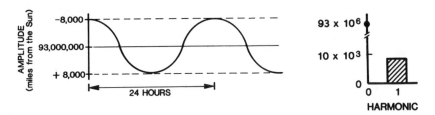

FIG 2–6.
Fourier (spectral) analysis of the distance from the sun to a point on the surface of the earth during a 24-hour period. On the left is the typical amplitude-time graph of the earth's motion. On the right is the Fourier spectrum, which is an amplitude-harmonic diagram. The amplitude diagram shows two values: a mean ("0" harmonic) distance of 93 million miles and a first (fundamental) harmonic distance of 8,000 miles. The first harmonic is at a frequency of 1/day.

nator, and the amplitude of the other harmonics is measured as a fraction of the first harmonic. The fraction may be greater or less than one; that is, the amplitude of higher harmonics is not constrained to have a lesser value than the fundamental, despite the importance we attach to its name. In general, the more rapidly moving and nonsinusoidal the appearance of the signal, the greater will be the level of the amplitude of the second and higher harmonics.

Relationship Between Spectral Analysis and Bandwidth.—The Fourier analysis of a signal allocates an amplitude and phase angle for a series of frequencies or harmonics of the signal, thereby weighting each according to its importance and timing. The bandwidth is a much simpler description of the signal and is derived from the spectral analysis. It is a continuous range of frequencies, unweighted in their relative amplitude or importance, which encompasses the frequency content of the Fourier spectrum.

Theoretically, the number of harmonics needed to characterize a periodic signal by spectral analysis is unlimited. That implies that there is no limit to the upper frequency of the bandwidth of a signal—it is infinite. This is where the relative amplitude of the harmonics is important. It turns out that, practically speaking, a small number of harmonics (no more than a few dozen for many biologic signals) are usually all that is necessary to characterize the signal, because the shape of many biologic waveforms is not that complex. This can be shown by inference, or by formal mathematical analysis.

We can determine bandwidth by inference from the spectral analysis. The information contained in the amplitude and phase from a limited number of harmonics of the spectral analysis is used to reconstruct a model of the original signal. The model is then compared to the original to see where and how much it deviates from the original. Harmonic terms are added or removed and the effect of this is judged visually. The bandwidth is then said to extend up to that harmonic (and its associated frequency) which appears to be visually important.

We can determine bandwidth by formal mathematical analysis of the spectral analysis by calculation of the variance ratio. The information contained in a cumulative series of harmonics from the spectral analysis is compared to the information contained in the original signal. Whereas increasing the number of harmonics always increases the quotient of this ratio, at some point in a series of harmonics the increase is very small. The bandwidth is then said to extend up to that harmonic (and its associated frequency) which meets some test or threshold value of added information.

Very Low Frequencies.—The Fourier spectrum or frequency spectrum gives the investigator a good idea of the high frequencies of the signal bandwidth, but not of the very low frequencies—the frequencies below the first harmonic. In the Fourier spectrum, low frequencies appear as part of the zeroth harmonic, which is also called the average or DC level of the signal. For reasons discussed above, it may not be appropriate or necessary to measure an average or DC level of the signal; also, the errors associated with some instruments may not permit the recording of a DC level (see *drift* in chapter 3). However, it may be appropriate and necessary to measure some very low frequencies that are a bit over zero frequency or near DC. Unfortunately, the frequency spectrum doesn't provide us with assistance in measuring this ultralow frequency content. The estimation of what is adequate with respect to signal frequency content and what is possible with respect to instrument bandwidth continues to be one of those unresolved areas of signal measurement. Later in this chapter, we'll have some practical advice on this problem.

Distortion due to Inadequate Bandwidth.—The result of using an instrument that has an inadequate bandwidth to capture the frequency response of the signal is distortion. An inadequate bandwidth or frequency response may occur because the instrument distorts the amplitude (either increases or decreases) or shifts the phase (alters the timing) of frequency components of the signal. A graphical display of a signal recorded by such an instrument would change the appearance of such a signal, and measurements obtained from the signal would not be correct. For example, the effects of using an instrument that did not have an adequate high-frequency response, because it reduced the amplitude of the high-frequency components of a signal, would be to "slow down" rapidly moving portions of the signal. Rapidly moving slopes and waves would be blunted and would appear to be moving more slowly. The effects of using an instrument that did not have an adequate low-frequency response, because it reduced the amplitude of the low-frequency components of a signal, would be to "speed up" slow-moving portions of the signal. Slowly moving slopes and steady portions of the signal would sag and appear to be changing. Inadequate frequency response of instruments is a form of nonrandom error, which is described further in chapter 3.

Frequency Content of Signals
Music.—An example of a spectral analysis of the waveforms of musical instruments is shown in Figure 2–7. I analyzed the musical

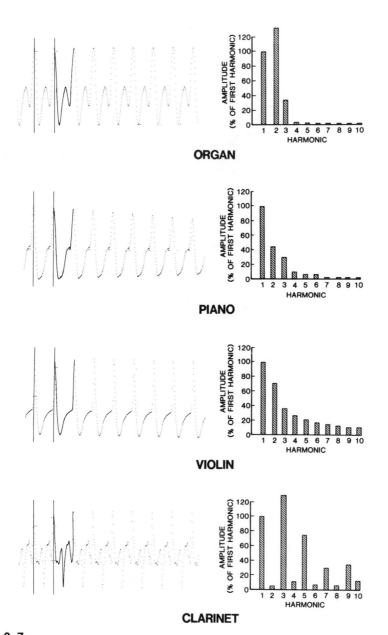

FIG 2–7.
Fourier (spectral) analysis of the sound of a musical note (the great octave "C") produced by four instruments. On the left is the amplitude-time diagram. The two vertical lines show the period of the signal (equivalent to a frequency of 65 Hz). One cycle of each note has

note called the great octave "C" (described earlier) for an organ, violin, piano, and clarinet.

Note that the spectral analysis or frequency content of each of the four instruments does not include a zero frequency term—the level of the mean or DC term is zero. Does that imply that there is no signal? No—it just means that the signal swings around a zero or DC level. The ultimate instrument used to detect musical signals is our ears. Because human audition does not have the capability of detecting frequencies below 20 Hz, we could not "hear" a DC or near DC frequency.

The spectral analysis does include a first harmonic, or fundamental, and a series of higher harmonics. The frequency of the first harmonic for each of the four instruments is 65.41 Hz, which is the definition of the tone called the great octave "C." The contrast among the notes of each instrument is the relative amplitude of the higher harmonics. The organ and the piano produce the simplest spectrum. That is, only a fundamental and a few additional harmonics have a substantial amplitude. The violin has a more complex spectrum, with additional harmonic terms. The clarinet is most intriguing, with its oscillating frequency spectrum. It is actually the variations in the amplitudes of these higher harmonics, these overtones, that give the musical instruments their distinctive sound quality, and provide the variation and the beauty we appreciate as music. To learn how we performed these spectral analyses on a computer, see chapter 8 ("Computers as Instruments").

The bandwidth would be obtained as follows: From visual inspection of the frequency spectra, I would estimate that the important harmonics of the great octave "C" for the organ and piano are up to six harmonics. Therefore, the bandwidth of this signal would be up to 390 Hz (6 × 65). The important harmonics for the violin and clarinet extend to at least ten harmonics. The bandwidth of this signal would be up to 650 Hz (10 × 65). An instrument that is used to measure these music signals would be required to have a bandwidth at least equal to that of the signal. To see what happens to the music signal from a clar-

---

been traced for emphasis. Note that although each instrument's note repeats itself exactly at a frequency of 65 Hz, there is considerable variation of the shape of the note among the instruments. On the right is the Fourier spectrum of one cycle, which is an amplitude-harmonic diagram. The zero frequency (mean) amplitude is zero, and is not shown. Note the variation of the first ten harmonics between the instruments. The harmonics in the spectrum represent the frequencies that are present in this periodic musical note. The differences in the amplitudes of the harmonics account for the complex shape of the waveforms and the distinct differences in sound of the instruments.

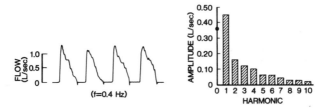

FIG 2–8.
Fourier (spectral) analysis of expiratory flow rate of a human. On the left is the amplitude-time diagram. The basic frequency of the signal is 0.4 Hz. On the right is the Fourier spectrum of one cycle of the signal. There is a zero frequency (mean) amplitude term, and a series of amplitudes of the first ten harmonic terms.

inet that is measured by a pen recorder with an inadequate frequency response, see Figure 7–2 in chapter 7.

Respiration.—The spectral analysis of the expiratory flow signal described previously in qualitative terms is shown in Figure 2–8. This spectral analysis includes a zero frequency or average term with an amplitude of 0.36 L/sec. The frequency of the first harmonic term is equal to the basic frequency of the flow signal (0.4 Hz). Note that its amplitude is more than the amplitude of the average term. The frequency of the additional harmonics are multiples of the fundamental. Note that their amplitude gradually declines. In order to use an instrument to measure this signal, it would have to have a bandwidth from DC to about 4 Hz (the frequency of the tenth harmonic). Note that if the absolute frequency of the fundamental changes, the frequency of the harmonics will also change, and this alters the bandwidth. For example, if the respiratory rate increases to 0.8 Hz, the bandwidth would increase to about 8 Hz.

Arterial and Pulmonary Artery Pressure.—The spectral analyses of the intravascular pressures that we described previously in qualitative terms are shown in Figure 2–9. The spectral analyses include a zero frequency or average term. For the arterial pressure, the amplitude of this term is about 48 mm Hg; for the pulmonary artery pressure, the amplitude of this term is about 8 mm Hg. The amplitude of the first harmonic (which has a frequency of 1.3 Hz) is considerably less than the average. The amplitudes of the first few harmonics rapidly decrease. In order to use an instrument to measure these pressure signals, it would have to have a bandwidth from DC to about 13 Hz (the frequency of the tenth harmonic). If the absolute frequency of the fundamental changes, the frequency of the harmonics also changes, and this would alter the bandwidth.

Estimating Signal Bandwidth

How does one obtain this vital information about the frequency content of a signal? Signals that have been studied previously may have had their frequency content analyzed, and it is incumbent on an investigator to dig out this information. Sometimes this information on frequency content is informally available by application of the "grand-

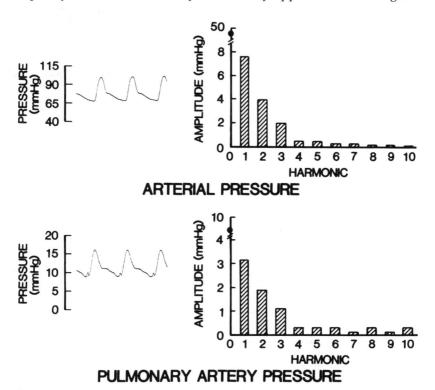

ARTERIAL PRESSURE

PULMONARY ARTERY PRESSURE

FIG 2–9.
Fourier (spectral) analysis of cardiovascular pressure signals. On the left is the almost periodic signal of arterial pressure *(top)* and pulmonary artery pressure *(bottom)*. The frequency of both is 1.3 Hz. On the right is the Fourier spectrum of one cycle of the signals. There is a zero frequency (mean) amplitude term, and a series of harmonics. Pressures in the arterial and pulmonary vascular beds are different, and therefore the amplitudes of the harmonics are different. The subtle differences of the shapes of the two waveforms are expressed as the relationship of the amplitude of the harmonics. Significant amplitudes out to about ten harmonics are present in both spectra; bandwidth would be from DC to about 13 Hz.

mother" principle *(I know exactly what my grandmother looks like, even if I can't express the exact rules for describing her)*; however, what everybody knows and accepts about bandwidth of a signal may not be correct. Some signals have not been so well studied.

Published Studies.—Careful reading of the experiments and publications of other investigators should reveal what they thought the frequency content of the signal under study was; unfortunately, few investigators bother to report such information. Also, some instruments have been designed to meet the bandwidth specifications of a particular signal. For example, advisory panels of physicians, scientists, and engineers have recommended that the human electrocardiograph (the instrument) should have a bandwidth from 0.05 Hz to 80 Hz. However, it really is obligatory for the investigator to match the specifications of the instrument with that of the signal.

Tables.—Table 2–1 allows you to look up the bandwidth of a limited selection of human signals. It is important to recognize the limitations of such tables. If we were to paint bandwidth with a broad brushstroke, we would conclude that the frequency content of biologic signals is from 0 to 20,000 Hz. However, this is much too broad a bandwidth—especially at the high-frequency end—for the vast majority of signals. General tables of signal bandwidth represent a compromise between what a reader wants to know "on the average" about signal bandwidth, and what circumstances govern alterations of signal bandwidth. This is important since there are real limitations of the frequency response of many instruments, whereas one would not unnecessarily want to prohibit signal measurement if an instrument had an adequate frequency response for the measurement.

There are a few questions one needs to ask about such a table. First, one needs to know for what species of biologic organism the table is providing data. Many tables don't state this critical information. For example, the frequency content of the arterial pressure of a human and a rat are substantially different (see below). Then, one needs to know the conditions under which the signal was analyzed for frequency content. For example, published tables of signal bandwidth from the cardiovascular and respiratory systems are usually based on a low fundamental frequency—the frequency of the system at rest. This might be 1.0 to 1.5 Hz for the cardiovascular system and 0.2 to 0.3 Hz in the respiratory system. However, under another condition—such as exercise—it is possible to have a two- to threefold increase of heart rate up to 3.5 Hz and a four- or fivefold increase of respiratory rate up to 1.5 Hz. This definitely changes signal bandwidth. Finally, one needs to know whether or not the information in the table is appropriate to the analysis or processing that is planned for the signal. I can cite two extremes of signal bandwidth. If it is planned to analyze the average of a signal, then (by definition) the frequency content of

TABLE 2–1.
Level and Bandwidth of Some Human Signals

SIGNAL	AMPLITUDE RANGE (HEALTH AND DISEASE)	FREQUENCY RANGE REQUIRED FOR GOOD MEASUREMENT (HZ)
CARDIOVASCULAR SYSTEM (Based on resting condition with a cardiac frequency of 1.5 Hz)		
Electrophysiology		
Body surface ECG	0 to 5 mV	0.05 to 80 Hz
Direct cardiac ECG	0 to 20 mV	0.05 to 80 Hz
His bundle electrogram	0 to 1 mV	30 to 300 Hz
Late potentials	0 to 20 μV	25 to 250 Hz
Pressure		
Arterial	20 to 300 mm Hg	0 to 15 Hz
Ventricular	−5 to 300 mm Hg	0 to 15 Hz
Differentiated arterial or ventricular	−2,000 to 3,000 mm Hg/sec	0 to 30 Hz
Venous	−5 to 30 mm Hg	0 to 10 Hz
Blood Flow		
Pulsatile cardiac output	0 to 1,000 ml/sec	0 to 15 Hz
Indicator dilution output	0 to 10 L/min	0 and near DC
Doppler flow velocity	0 to 5 m/sec	0 to 15 Hz
Limb plethysmography	Variable	0 to 5 Hz
Phonocardiography	80 dB	20 to 300 Hz
RESPIRATORY SYSTEM (Based on resting condition with a respiratory frequency of 0.3 Hz)		
Respiratory function		
Flow rate	0 to 2 L/sec	0 to 5 Hz
Body plethysmography	Variable	0 to 5 Hz
Blood gases and pH		
P_{O_2} (arterial and venous)	10 to 650 mm Hg	0 to 2 Hz
P_{CO_2} (as above)	10 to 90 mm Hg	0 to 2 Hz
PCO (as above)	0 to 75 mm Hg	0 to 2 Hz
pH (as above)	6.9 to 7.7 pH	0 to 2 Hz
Diffusing capacity (CO)	16 to 35 ml CO/mm Hg/min	0 to 2 Hz

(continued)

TABLE 2–1. *Continued*

SIGNAL	AMPLITUDE RANGE (HEALTH AND DISEASE)	FREQUENCY RANGE REQUIRED FOR GOOD MEASUREMENT (HZ)
NEUROMUSCULAR SYSTEM (Based on resting condition)		
Electroencephalography		
Body surface	5 to 300 μV	0.2 to 50 Hz
Brain surface	10 to 5000 μV	0.2 to 50 Hz
Evoked potentials	0 to 50 μV	10 to 500 Hz
Electromyography	0.1 to 5 mV	20 to 2,500 Hz
Eye potentials		
Electroretinogram	0 to 1000 μV	0 to 20 Hz
Electro-oculogram	50 to 5000 μV	0.2 to 15 Hz
GASTROINTESTINAL AND UROLOGICAL SYSTEMS		
Gastrointestinal mechanics		
Pressure	0 to 100 cm H_2O	0 to 10 Hz
Force	1 to 50 gm	0 to 1 Hz
Electrogastrogram		
Skin surface	10 to 1,000 μV	0.05 to 1 Hz
Stomach surface	0.5 to 80 mV	0.05 to 1 Hz
Bladder pressure	0 to 100 cm H_2O	0 to 10 Hz
MISCELLANEOUS BIOMEDICAL SIGNALS		
Core temperature	20 to 42° C	0 and near DC
Galvanic skin response	1 to 500 kOhm	0.1 to 1 Hz
Voice	0 to 100 dB	20 to 20,000 Hz
Displacement, velocity acceleration	Variable	Variable
Chemical chromatograms	Variable	Typically < 75 Hz

the signal is DC. On the other hand, if it is planned to analyze the differential of a signal, then the frequency content includes higher frequencies than are usually required for an adequate measurement of the signal itself (see chapter 6, "Signal Processors").

Under some circumstances, it may be appropriate to estimate the bandwidth of a signal based on extrapolation from published tables. For example, the most important phenomenon that changes signal frequency content in the cardiovascular and respiratory systems is the basic frequency of the signal. Table 2–1 shows a frequency content for arterial pressure of up to 15 Hz based on a fundamental frequency of up to 1.5 Hz. If the fundamental frequency increases to 3 Hz, then a reasonable extrapolation of the signal bandwidth would be up to 30 Hz. However, it is also possible that the shape of the signal changes because of changes of the way in which the heart develops pressure or the vascular system alters its properties. In that case, extrapolation of signal bandwidth may not be appropriate.

As another example of extrapolation, it is reasonable to consider that most mammalian species are constructed similarly and only the fundamental frequency of their systems (cardiovascular, respiratory, etc.) is different between systems. The heart rate of an anesthetized rat is about 6 Hz, and the frequency content of the arterial pressure is up to 50 Hz. This is very close to what would be anticipated by extrapolation from the bandwidth of human arterial pressure. I've personally verified this for arterial pressure signals in animals from humans down to rats, and the available literature supports this concept for the cardiovascular system of most mammals used in laboratory investigations. I am not aware of a comprehensive body of literature that would allow extrapolation to other systems between species.

Table 2–1 may be incomplete for your needs, and information from the literature may not be readily available. You then need to perform a spectral analysis to obtain the data. This is possible to do with equipment designed for this purpose (spectrum analyzer), and all students should work through this route conceptually. In reality, you need some heuristics (rules of thumb) for estimating bandwidth. The following is an eyeball method: you're going to use your eyes to pick out those parts of the signal that are at the extremes of the bandwidth. This method still requires some instrumentation, but it's not as intractable as analysis of the frequency spectrum.

High-Frequency Content.—The concept of this technique is to estimate the highest frequency of the bandwidth based on the *fastest moving* part of the signal. You need to use some equipment that has a bandwidth in excess of (your guess) as to the high-frequency content of the signal, and some method of measuring the duration of the fastest moving part of the signal. The preferred choice is a wide bandwidth amplifier and storage oscilloscope—one that will temporarily hold the tracing on its screen. These instruments should be available in an instrumentation shop or engineering facility (often called the "clinical engineering" department in a hospital). A second choice is a wide bandwidth instrumentation amplifier linked to a light (or UV) writing recorder. These instruments should be available in someone's laboratory.

The process of estimating high-frequency content is to record the signal and measure the duration of the fastest rising or falling part of the signal (Fig 2–10). You must make sure that you clearly can see the

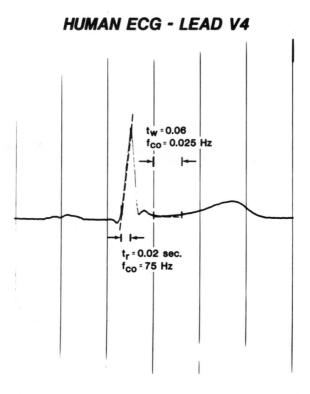

HUMAN ECG - LEAD V4

$t_w = 0.06$
$f_{co} = 0.025$ Hz

$t_r = 0.02$ sec.
$f_{co} = 75$ Hz

FIG 2–10.
Estimating signal bandwidth. The extremes of frequency content—the high and the low frequencies—depend on the rapid and slow-moving parts of the signal, respectively. Here, an estimation is made of the bandwidth of a surface ECG signal. The duration of the most rapid and the slowest parts of the signal are measured, and the bandwidth estimated from formulas suggested in the text.

beginning and the end of the most rapid event, and that you can measure its duration. This usually means running the recorder or the oscilloscope at very high speed in order to gain enough time resolution to perform this. From the measured duration of the most rapid event, one calculates the highest frequency in the signal. A stringent formula for this high frequency (f_h, Hz) is:

$$f_h = 1.5/t_{r \text{ or } f}$$

where $t_{r \text{ or } f}$ is the duration of the maximum rise- or falltime component in the signal in seconds. This frequency will correspond to a "cutoff" of negligible distortion from an engineering point of view (see "Filters" in chapter 6) and no visible waveform change. A less stringent requirement will take two thirds of this value. This is the "cutoff" for acceptable distortion of the signal—that is, no visual risetime degradation, but some rounding of abrupt changes.

Low-Frequency Content.—The concept of this technique is to estimate the lowest frequency of the bandwidth from the *slowest moving* part of the signal. The slowest moving part is a flat or unchanging part of the signal, and the object is to measure the duration of the longest unchanging portion of the signal (see Fig 2–10). The requirements for the instruments needed to measure the low-frequency content again must equal or exceed (the expected) low-frequency response of the signal. This is best performed with a DC coupled amplifier, or if the signal has drift or bias that must be blocked in order to be recorded, an ultra-low AC coupled amplifier. The recorder or display requirements are less demanding since most devices can record down to DC. However, the speed and resolution of the recording must be sufficient to measure accurately the duration of the flat portion of the signal.

The process of estimating the lowest frequency is to record the signal and measure the duration of an unchanging part of the signal. You must make sure that you clearly can see the beginning and the end of this part of the signal, and that you can measure its duration. A stringent formula for low-frequency content (f_l, Hz) is:

$$f_l = 0.0016/t_w$$

where t_w is the duration of the longest flat portion of the signal in seconds. This frequency will correspond to the cutoff of the signal where there will be negligible distortion. A less stringent requirement is five times this value. This is the cutoff required for slight visible degradation of the signal.

As a very rough rule of thumb, the lowest frequency component of a biologic signal is about 1/20th of the fundamental frequency. You'll recall that the fundamental frequency of a periodic signal was equal to the basic period of the signal, and the low frequency component will be about 1/20th of that. For example, most cardiac events have a fundamental frequency equal to that of the heartbeat, about 1 Hz (60 per minute) in the resting human. Our rule of thumb would recommend that, if we can't use an amplifier with a frequency response down to 0 Hz (DC), we should anticipate recording low-frequency components down to 0.05 Hz.

3

Measurement Theory and Instrument Errors

Measurement is the assignment of numbers
to objects or events according to rules.
S. S. Stevens

Having gotten this far in the book, the reader may want to ask, "Why should I study about instrumentation?" There are many cooks who can produce a tasty cake, yet they understand little about the composition of cake ingredients and the thermodynamic and chemical processes that occur during baking. If you are of this sort, you have my blessing to read no further. However, the theory and practice of instrumentation have advanced so far and so rapidly—something we really could not say for cake baking—that it is plausible to entertain the thought that long-term benefit may accrue from an understanding of the foundations of the theory and practice of instrumentation.

WHAT YOU NEED TO KNOW

1. Instrumentation science and measurement theory are the practical and theoretical branches of measurement science. Two important concepts—truth and consistency—are common to both fields and share the same definition, but the terms used may vary.

2. Measurement theory provides the basis for consideration of error which is an inherent part of the process of measurement. There are two types of error: nonrandom and random. These error types influence our confidence in the truth and consistency of our observations, respectively.

3. Performance characteristics—called *specifications*—describe the operation and limitation of operation of instruments, including the types and amounts of error.

Measurement Science

Instrumentation science and measurement theory are the empirical and theoretical branches, respectively, of measurement science. Both are usually considered part of the larger discipline of information science, which includes such high-flying fields as computer science, mathematics (including statistics), communications, and cybernetics. Many of the terms used in these fields have common definitions, even though the nomenclature of the terms is different. Of greatest importance, the terms we will encounter in this chapter deal with the *truth* of the observation of a signal and the *consistency* of the observation of a signal.

Truth relates to how closely the observed signal adheres to a "gold standard" or represents the underlying concept of what is being measured. The terms used to express this definition are *accuracy* and *validity* in instrumentation science and measurement theory, respectively. *Consistency* relates to how reproducibly the observation of the signal yields the same results on repeated observation. The terms used to express this definition are *precision* and *reliability* in instrumentation science and measurement theory, respectively (Table 3–1).

It makes no sense to observe a biologic signal by use of an instrument unless (1) the observer can be confident that the observed signal is what was intended to convey the information about the biologic phe-

TABLE 3–1.
Terms Used in Measurement Theory and Instrumentation Science

	SOURCE OF ERROR	MEASUREMENT OF ERROR
	TRUTH	
Measurement theory	Nonrandom	Validity
Instrumentation science	Bias	Accuracy
	CONSISTENCY	
Measurement theory	Random	Reliability
Instrumentation science	Noise	Precision

nomenon—that is, it is true—and (2) unless the observation could be repeated and yield the same results—that is, it is consistent. However, things are not always as they should be, and all measurements, including those made by an instrument, have some limitations or *errors.*

Measurement Theory

The Concept of Error

Fundamental to measurement theory is the concept of error. The goal of error-free measurement is never achieved in any area of scientific investigation. *Error is what defines the level of confidence we have in both the validity (truth) and reliability (consistency) of our observations.* When error associated with validity is small, then we are confident about the validity or truth of our signal observation, and vice versa. When error associated with reliability is low, then we are confident about the reliability or consistency of our signal observation, and vice versa. This can be expressed as follows:

$$x = T + (E_v + E_r)$$

or, the observed measurement *(x)* is the sum of the true value of the measurement *(T)* plus the errors. The error associated with validity (E_v) is called *nonrandom* or *systematic error,* and the error associated with reliability (E_r) is called *random error* or *noise.* In the scheme of biologic measurements, the locus or place of measurement error can occur either at the source of the signal, in the instruments, or at the ports or connections between these two.

Nonrandom Error

Nonrandom error or bias is a systematic or consistent form of error that causes the observed measurement to deviate from the true measurement in a reproducible or predictable manner. The level of nonrandom error determines our level of confidence in the validity of our observations. All instruments have systematic error or bias, and this determines our confidence in the accuracy of the instruments to assist us in these observations. The types of nonrandom errors found in instruments are discussed in the next section.

Random Error

Random error is an unpredictable form of error that causes an inconstant amount and direction of deviation from the true measurement during any single observation, the average deviation of which tends toward zero as the number of repeated observations of the same phenomenon increases. The level of random error determines our level of confidence in the reliability of our observations. All instruments have random errors, and this determines our confidence in the precision of the instruments to assist us in these observations. The types of random errors found in instruments are discussed in the next section.

Reducing the Effects of Error

The practical application of measurement theory is to recognize the types and amounts of error during observation of the biologic signal. Under some circumstances, it may be possible to limit the amount of error during observation and thereby improve our confidence in the observed measurement. To reduce the amount of error due to an instrument, the experimenter has two choices: (1) devise a new instrument that has a reduced amount of error, or (2) deal with the types of error presented by the current instrumentation.

Examples of the former are legion in the 20th century. Scientists have repeatedly abandoned older instruments that had a large degree of error in favor of those with a lesser degree of error. It is also possible to limit the error without abandoning the instruments at hand. The experimenter limits the effects of nonrandom error by recognizing the types of systematic error or bias that are present in the instrumentation system, and by performing a *calibration*. The information learned from calibration may be used to reduce the amount of error either before or after the observation. The experimenter limits the effects of random error by *increasing the number of observations of the signal and averaging those observations* so as to reduce the effect of the deviations. The effects of random error decrease in proportion to the square root of the number of observations that are averaged.

Specification of Instrument Error

There are a number of characteristics that define the operation—and limitation—of instruments. These *performance characteristics* are so important that they have been universally recognized and adopted into a formal nomenclature of instrument characteristics called *specifications*. We will encounter a variety of instrument specifications throughout the book. Here, we will discuss specifications that have to do with instrument error.

Accuracy

Accuracy is the instrumentation science version of *truth*, which is the ability of the instrument to measure faithfully the true or correct level (amount, quantity, or characteristics) of the signal.or to represent the underlying concept of the system under study. In the application of instrumentation, the experimenter grapples with two limitations to accuracy: *biologic* and *instrumental*. At times it is difficult to distinguish between these limitations.

The first limitation is whether the observed signal represents the underlying biologic concept that the experimenter wanted to study. Suppose we are interested in studying pulmonary function. As described in chapter 2, we have a few choices to consider in the study of any biologic system: structure, function, and biochemistry are but a few possibilities. Are we confident that the signal we have chosen to measure (such as airflow, mechanics, or blood gases) represents the concept of lung function? As has happened commonly during the last century, a new variable is discovered that could be an additional or even preferred signal to study, which would characterize lung function. We might have to revise or even abandon our current instruments in favor of new ones in order to increase our confidence in the accuracy of our observations. It is worth applying a considerable amount of thought to this matter, because once an investigation of a particular signal is launched, it develops a life of its own with a substantial commitment of time, effort, money, and investigator ego.

The second limitation is that imposed by the instrumentation. Once the investigator has determined which is the most accurate signal to observe, it is important to use an instrument that has *selectivity*. This is the ability of an instrument to identify correctly the signal under study and to distinguish this signal from other signals. In the previous chapter, we pointed out that there were a large number of biologic signal sources, but only a limited number of different signal characteristics. The investigator may only be interested in the EEG, but bioelectrical signals are also generated in the heart, skeletal muscles, and nerves. In addition to distinguishing among these different biologic signals, it is also necessary for the instrument to distinguish the EEG from nonspecific electrical noise or interference.

Once having chosen a system to study, having developed confidence that a particular signal represents the underlying concept, and having chosen an instrument that is selective, one considers the accuracy of the instrument to measure the signal of interest. Let's review some of the nonrandom errors that are associated with limitation of accuracy (Fig 3–1).

Offset Error.—The offset error or bias error is a constant level of error that either adds to or subtracts from the true measurement re-

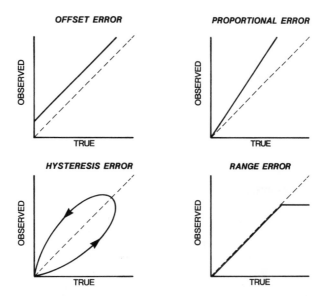

FIG 3–1.
Nonrandom errors. Four different types of errors are shown—offset, proportional, hysteresis, and range.

gardless of the level of the measurement (see Fig 3–1). If positive, the offset adds to the true measurement, and therefore the observed measurement is higher than the truth. If negative, the offset subtracts from the true measurement, and therefore the observed measurement is lower than the truth. For example, a weighing scale with no weight applied might read below zero, say −5 lb (the dream of every dieter). Then all observed measurements of weight will show a systematic bias and will be reduced by 5 lb compared to the true weight.

Drift Error.—The drift error is a time-dependent form of offset error in which offset is minimal to begin with, and progressively increases or increases to a maximum over some period of time. It is also possible for drift to occur first in one direction, then another. Drift is considered to be a slowly occurring phenomenon or, more precisely, a low-frequency event below 0.1 Hz. Higher frequency forms of drift are called *noise*. Some forms of noise have random characteristics and are considered under random error.

Proportional Error.—This systematic error is in proportion to the level of the measurement. The simplest type of proportional error will be linearly proportional—that is, the error will be a percentage of the level of the measurement (see Fig 3–1). However, more complex types of proportional errors are possible in which the error is predictable, but nonlinear, according to the level of the measurement. Again, the proportional error may be positive or negative with respect to the level of the measurement. For example, a weighing scale may have a linearly proportional error of $+10\%$. A true weight of 10 lb will become an observed measurement of 11 lb. A true weight of 100 lb will become an observed measurement of 110 lb. Proportional and offset errors may occur independently or together.

History Dependency (Hysteresis) Error.—This systematic error is dependent on the previous level of the measurement; that is, the current observation is based on the true value plus some value determined by the preceding history of measurements. The amount of error that occurs may be different when the history of the measurement goes from lower to higher levels, from when the history of measurement goes from higher to lower levels. History errors may be all positive, all negative, or a mixture of positive and negative values. Both electrical (particularly electromagnetic) and mechanical devices and components are prone to hysteresis errors.

For example, a weighing scale could contain a spring as the critical component for weight determination. If 100 lb is placed on the scale it might be observed to weigh 95 lb, and one might guess that either an offset or a proportional error has occurred. However, without removing this weight, an additional 100 lb is added and the true and observed weight are both, say, 200 lb. Strange scale, you say. But even stranger, the second 100 lb is removed (leaving the first 100 lb on the scale) and the observed measurement is 105 lb. That is, the errors that influenced the true measurement of 100 lb depended on whether a higher or lower level of weight was on the scale before the measurement. It is possible to misclassify this form of error as random, unless a careful review of the history of the observations is made.

Range Error.—This systematic error occurs when the true measurement is outside of the useful measurement range of the instrument. All physical devices have limitations with respect to the range of observations they can report. If this range is exceeded, then error may occur. One type of this error is clipping or overrange. That is, even though the true measurement increases, the observed measurement remains at a lower level—the instrument can't report a higher value. The opposite can also occur: clipping due to underrange, where the true measurement decreases below the range that can be observed.

A more subtle and devastating form of range error occurs when the bounds of the useful range are exceeded, and an error less obvious than clipping occurs, such as a proportional or hysteresis error. A third possible subtype of range error would be a catastrophic failure mode: the instrument breaks, the scale reports either no value or a wild range of values, and the instrument is found to be inoperable. For example, a weighing instrument has a range of 0 to 200 lb and small systematic errors within this range. A weight of 300 lb is placed on the scale, and the scale still reads 200 lb (clipping of observed measurement), or perhaps 250 lb (introduction of a large error), or perhaps the dial spins around and the scale can no longer be used (broken).

Scale Error.—This systematic error is an error that occurs during the reading of a scale or marking device that displays the level of the measurement. Most scale errors occur when an observed measurement falls in between the defined, known, or marked measuring values of which an instrument is capable of reporting. The resolving power—the ability to measure finer and finer parts of the level of the measurement—is limited by both the conceptual and physical principles of the instrument. When an observed value falls between two scale markings, a scale error may occur.

One form of scale error is *truncation*, in which any additional level of the signal that falls between two scale markings is eliminated, and the level of the measurement assumes the next *lower* level for which there is a scale marking. This results in a systematic underestimation of the level of the signal. Another form of scale error is *rounding*, in which any additional level of the signal that falls between two scale markings is rounded to the nearest scale marking. This results in a systematic underestimation of some signals, and a systematic overestimation of others.*

For completeness, it is worthwhile adding to this list scale reading errors due to parallax, in which the reading is taken from a line of sight that is nonperpendicular to the pointer and the scale. The line of sight then causes alignment of the pointer with an incorrect scale value. This observed level is usually systematically either higher or lower than the true level of the signal, but a random error could result.

---

*It is arguable whether this should be classified as nonrandom or random error. *Interpolation*, another form of scale error related to rounding, is classified as a random error and is discussed later in the chapter.

For example, a weighing instrument has a graticule (scale marking device) that is marked in increments of 1 lb. Let's say that true weights of either 47.3 or 47.8 lb are placed on the instrument, which causes the scale pointer to fall somewhere between the 47 and the 48 lb mark. If the instrument had a truncation error, then the level of the observed measurement would be reported as 47 lb for either of the two weights. If the instrument had a rounding error, then a true weight of 47.3 lb would be reported as 47 lb, while a true weight between 47.8 lb would be reported as 48 lb.

Frequency Response Error.—This error occurs whenever the level of a signal is modified (either increased or decreased) according to its frequency, or when the phase relationship among the frequencies is modified from their actual relationship. This causes a distortion of a signal, which means that there will be errors in the level or the timing of the signal or both.

As detailed in chapter 2, it is very important to match the bandwidth of the instrument to the frequency content of the signal and the intended analysis of the signal. The bandwidth or frequency response of an instrument is that interval of frequencies over which there is accurate and precise measurement of the level and phase of the signal frequencies. The instrument should accurately measure the amplitude (level) of each frequency component of the signal, and the instrument should cause no phase shift among the frequency components.

Resonance and attenuation are especially interesting distortions of the bandwidth that can occur in many instruments, but which frequently are present in instruments that contain mechanical components, such as strain gauge transducers (chapter 5) and recorders (chapter 7). All instruments draw some energy from the signal source at the input to the instrument. The amount of energy absorbed from the signal must be minimized to avoid attenuating (decreasing) the actual level of the signal. Of equal importance, the level of energy absorbed should be constant across the bandwidth.

Resonance occurs when the instrument gives back at some band of frequencies some of this absorbed energy (Fig 3–2). The result is that the instrument increases the level of the signal above 100% of its value at lower frequencies, sometimes to a substantially increased level. This is a form of amplification that is dependent on frequency, and although there are rare and important exceptions in the design of instruments, resonance is usually considered undesirable. Attenuation is the opposite phenomenon: the instrument absorbs additional energy at some band of frequencies beyond that absorbed at others. The result is a decrease in amplitude of the signal below 100% of its level at lower frequencies, sometimes to a substantially reduced level.

If the amplitudes of the frequencies that compose the bandwidth of the signal are not measured accurately, there will be a distortion of the signal, which is a change of shape of the signal. This distortion may cause the peak amplitude of the signal to either increase (if resonance occurs) or decrease (if attenuation occurs). Additionally, the details of the shape of the waveform of the signal will be altered. Because instruments are constructed of physical components, it is not possible to have an infinitely flat bandwidth—that is, one that avoids resonance and attenuation. The point in the bandwidth of an instrument where the frequency response departs from the flat portion is called the *natural frequency*. It is necessary to use an instrument only over the flat

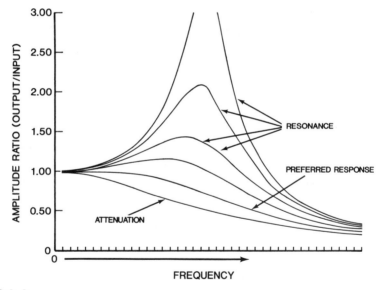

FIG 3–2.

Errors of frequency response—resonance and attenuation. Physical limitations in the construction of many instruments limit the useful frequency response of the instrument. One of the predictable errors is a change in the level of the signal over a range of frequencies that compose the signal. When resonance occurs, the level of the signal for those frequencies beyond the natural frequency actually increases. When attenuation occurs, the level of the signal for those frequencies beyond the natural frequency actually decreases. Because limitation of frequency response is unavoidable, most instruments are designed to optimize the band of frequencies where the level of the signal will be little changed. Such a design (indicated in the diagram as the *preferred response*) occurs in instruments that have been critically damped—that is, where resonance has been avoided and attenuation has been moved to higher frequencies.

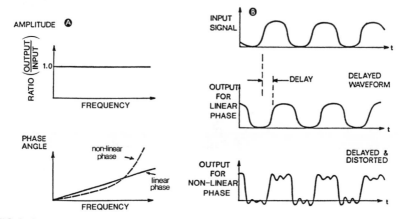

FIG 3–3.
Errors of frequency response—linear and nonlinear phase. Physical limitations in the construction of many instruments limit the useful frequency response of the instrument. One of the predictable errors is an alteration in the timing relationship among the various frequency components *(panel A)*.

portion of the bandwidth by limiting its use to signals whose bandwidth falls below the natural frequency.

Another type of frequency response error is altered phase relationship, which means that the timing relationship of the various frequencies of the bandwidth is changed. In the simplest form of phase error, the phase is shifted linearly with the frequency. This type of error is very frequent and sometimes acceptable because it does not distort the shape of the waveform of the signal, but merely causes a timing delay (Fig 3–3). However, if there is a nonlinear error in the phase relationship, the result is a delay and distortion of the waveform, which is usually not acceptable.

Precision

Precision is the instrument science version of the consistency of measurement. There are two aspects to signal precision: biologic precision and instrument precision. *Biologic precision* reflects the consistency or reproducibility of the level (amount, quantity, or characteristics) of the biologic event. *Instrumental precision* reflects the consistency or reproducibility of the instrument to measure the level of the biologic signal. It may be difficult to distinguish whether biologic or instrumental errors contribute to the limitation of precision of signal measurement.

Is it reasonable to expect that biologic behavior will be consistent?

The behavior of my 9-year-old son aside, biologic behavior in general has limited precision. Are heart rate and respiratory rate constant? Are the magnitude of blood pressure, tidal volume, and membrane depolarization constant? Some degree of biologic variation is expected and, in general, biologic variation is usually smaller within a subject or experimental preparation than it is between subjects or experimental preparations. The experimenter is commonly interested in trying to alter the behavior or seeking to observe altered behavior of the biologic system in order to learn what laws govern the system. Statistical tests used to detect differences are based on comparing the observed difference of the signal between states or conditions to the normally occurring variation of the signal.

The other source of limited precision is to be found in the instruments themselves. Let's review some of the random errors that are associated with limitation of instrument precision.

Noise.—This random error changes the level of any single observation in an unpredictable way. However, the average deviation over a very large (theoretically infinite) series of measurements is expected to be zero. Some of the sources of random error in instruments are caused by the heating of electrical or mechanical components, the presence of stray and unpredictable signals and energies in the environment, the alteration in the power supply that energizes the instrument, and the insecure mechanical connections between or within components.

Sometimes it is difficult to distinguish random from systematic errors, especially when the latter are multifaceted. For example, an observer would have great difficulty distinguishing hysteresis from random error, unless a series of pilot observations of types of error were made. Noise may affect instrument function in a particular way, as cited in the following examples.

Amplitude Linearity Error.—This error causes a variation of the output of the signal depending on the level of input. However, it is different from the previously mentioned *proportional error* in that the deviation of the output is not systematic. A simple measure of the error of amplitude linearity is made by observing the largest deviation of the output signal from what would have been predicted from a linear relationship between input and output. A more sophisticated determination of amplitude linearity error is called total harmonic distortion. It is made by measuring the output level to input level relationship of the instrument over its range, calculating a mathematical formula that approximates this relationship (called a power series), and calculating a type of RMS value from the ratio of the power series to a linear output-to-input relationship.

For example, the observed measurements of weight on a weighing scale are slightly larger or slightly smaller than the true weight over the range of the scale. The maximum deviation observed over this range is ±1 lb. A careful analysis of the observed to true measurements of the scale shows a 1% total harmonic distortion, which means that the RMS of the average deviation of measurement will be ±1% of the true measurement.

Range and Scale Error.—In the preceding section on instrument accuracy, we alluded to a number of types of error that are predominantly nonrandom, but could include some aspect of randomness. This duality of types of error also can occur in range and scale errors.

For example, when a range is exceeded it is possible for the instrument to report a random level, rather than reporting a level equal to the range limit. While it is true that many scale errors are nonrandom, *rounding and interpolation* are types of random scale error. When a level falls between two scale values, the observer may either round or interpolate between the values. In rounding, the observer chooses either of the two nearest scale markings. For example, a weighing instrument has a graticule that is marked in increments of 1 lb. A true weight of 47.5 lb is placed on the scale which causes the scale pointer to fall somewhere between the 47 and the 48 lb marks. The observed measurement might be recorded as either 47 or 48 lb, or a value might be interpolated.

The object of interpolation is to reduce the variation of the level of the measurement, but there is some randomness in the way in which the observer assigns this level such that it might be slightly lower or slightly higher than the true value. The true level, or an observation either higher or lower than the true level, might be made. Given experience and perhaps some encouragement by the way in which the scale is constructed, the investigator is likely to interpolate a true weight of 47.5 lb to a level of 47.4, 47.5, or 47.6 lb in an entirely random way. When rounding and interpolation are nonrandom, they result in the types of errors described previously.

Coping With Instrument Error

It is very important to obtain an estimate of the amount of both random and systematic error before making observations. This is useful both for biologic and for instrument errors. This is done by reviewing what information has been developed a priori on the errors in the system and by performing a calibration. I make additional comments about calibration in chapter 9, "Running the Experiment," but here we will focus the discussion on error specifications provided with an instrument.

Error specifications supplied with an instrument are in themselves a study in accuracy and precision. When a manufacturer makes a statement that ". . . both the accuracy and precision of this widget are ±1%," one needs to question where these data came from, particularly what calibration was performed to certify this level of error. The ultimate calibration of the instrument can be no better than the precision and accuracy of the known standard used for calibration. In addition, the error specifications should be qualified by additional specifications that characterize the operation of the instrument. The usual qualifiers for accuracy and precision are (1) the range or the level of the signal, and (2) the operating and environmental conditions.

Specification for Accuracy.—The specification for accuracy is usually dependent on the range of the instrument. Generally, two types of ranges will be specified: an operating range, and an overrange without failure range. It is the former range that usually qualifies statements of precision and accuracy. The range of an instrument should be thought of as both its capabilities to measure the level of static signals and, if intended to measure dynamic signals, its bandwidth. Usually much greater error accompanies an overrange compared to an operating range. When there is more than one operating range, there may be different error specifications for each range. If an instrument measures a continuous range of values, a typical specification for accuracy might be ± "x"% of the observed value. If an instrument measures a discrete range of values (such as seen on the scale markings of a recorder or the digits of a numerical display device), a typical specification for accuracy might be ± "x" digits or scale marks.

For example, a weighing instrument may have two operating ranges. For the operating range of 0 to 100 lb, the specification for precision and accuracy could be ±1% or ±1 lb. A second operating range of 0 to 10 lb may be accompanied by a specification of ±1% or ±0.1 lb. It is common for the percentage figure to be constant across ranges, while the absolute amount varies. This usually occurs when only the scale of an instrument is changed to alter the range of operation. When multiple components of an instrument are used to effect different ranges, it is likely that both the percentage and absolute level of accuracy will change.

Specification for Precision.—The specification for precision usually depends on the level of the signal. Noise, which is one of the major random errors, usually has a known range under specified conditions of operation. Because much of noise is 60 Hz interference from power mains, it is commonly expressed as an equivalent RMS value of voltage of the output of the instrument. As an alternative, precision may be reported as a percentage of noise to signal—for example, "x"% of a certain level of signal output from the instrument. Manufacturers usually calculate this quotient from the *maximum* signal output level that can be observed in a range of operation. It should be appreciated that the precision, when presented as a percentage, will usually be worse when one works with a signal that is at a low level of the range.

Specifications That Qualify Error Specifications.—The additional specifications that always qualify those for error are those for the operating and environmental conditions. These may include the temperature and relative humidity of the ambient air around the instrument, the characteristics of the voltage level and frequency (if AC) of the electrical power supplied to the instrument, and the time alloted for warm-up of the instrument. These specifications for operation should be appropriate for the conditions intended. For example, one could not hope to achieve the stated precision and accuracy of a recorder with ambient temperature specifications for operation of 5 to 30° C in an open field in Antarctica during the winter or the Sahara during the summer.

4

Instrumentation Theory and Practice

I suspect that most readers picked up this book for what is yet to come, rather than what already was. Your patience will be rewarded shortly: the meat and potatoes of the book come next. Permit me one additional indulgence as we provide the conceptual and practical basis for the usage of instruments.

WHAT YOU NEED TO KNOW

1. Collection of biologic data (observations) may be performed without instrumentation. Instrumentation is used either to amplify, detect, retain, or process observations beyond that of human capacity.

2. The process of measurement requires limiting the application of instruments to a defined biologic system, and measuring one or more aspects of the behavior (response) of that system in response to a naturally occurring or provoked stimulus without interfering with the operation of that system.

3. The science of instrumentation involves the concepts of observation, communication and control. The types of devices that demon-

strate these qualities are measurement aides, communication devices, and regulating and following devices (servomechanisms).

4. An instrument is capable of performing only a single function. To optimize the processes of observation, communication, and regulation, it is advantageous to configure multiple instruments together in a series and series-parallel manner of individual elements.

Decision to Use an Instrument

Why Use an Instrument?

The need for instrumentation arises from the need to convert a biologic signal into either a larger or more readily understood form than exists in nature, or to assist and extend the retention (memory or storage) and processing of that signal by the observer. The first step is to decide whether an instrument is needed.

Sometimes a biologic signal can be observed without the need for a measuring instrument, or a very simple instrument can be used. For example, the cardiac apical impulse sometimes can be observed by the eye or felt by the hand, and this observation can be clinically useful. The key to the possibility of such observations rests on (1) the transmission of the signal to the surface of the body, and (2) the ability to perceive the signal by one of the five human senses. Even if such observations are possible, it may be desirable to obtain additional information by supplementing the senses by instrumentation.

Simple Instruments.—For example, although the concept of arterial pressure existed prior to the 17th century by observation of spurting blood during a hemorrhage and by tactile examination of the peripheral pulses, additional information was provided by Stephen Hales when he exposed the femoral artery of a horse and directly connected the artery to a glass measuring tube; the height to which the tube filled with blood was a quantitative measurement of the arterial pressure. Further information about the arterial pressure was obtained by Ludwig during the 19th century when he connected an artery to a mercury column that had a float and writing lever at its top. The motion of the lever was transcribed onto a smoked drum, which allowed observation and preservation of the phasic aspects of the arterial pressure.

In clinical practice, venous pressure measurements are still made by visual observation of the height of the column of blood in the jugular vein. When more precise estimates were needed, it was still common practice a decade ago to measure central venous pressure by application of Hale's principle to a central vein—an example of the use of a simple instrument. More elaborate catheters, transducers, amplifiers, and recording instruments have been introduced only recently into routine clinical medicine.

Advanced Instruments.—Sometimes the signal cannot be detected by one of the five senses or even by simple instruments. Bioelectrical events were not suspected in excitable tissue until Galvani applied a small voltage to muscle and observed a muscle twitch. The proof that intrinsic electrical events caused muscle contraction awaited the more refined development of the galvanometer for the observation of the muscle action potential. Therefore the experimentalist is always balancing the characteristics of the signal with the questions to be addressed about the signal and the availability of instrumentation to assist the observation.

Efficiency and Economic Utility.—A crude or simple instrument may be satisfactory because its efficiency is high, even when it is recognized that the information obtained about the biologic signal is limited. I would define the efficiency of an instrument in terms of its practical and economic utility: it is the quotient of information obtained divided by the effort and cost expended in application. The cost and difficulty in implementing some instruments may be so large that their use may be obviated. Society is currently debating the merits of some expensive and widely duplicated biomedical instruments. The debate is worthwhile; however, objections are suspended by anyone who witnessed the replacement of the inexpensive (but virtually medieval) neurodiagnostic procedure called a pneumoencephalogram, in favor of the expensive technology of the CT scan.

Concepts in Application of Instruments

The System to Be Measured

In defining what signal it is that you wish to measure, one is actually recognizing and defining the existence of a *system* that emits that signal, and distinguishing that system from the rest of the world.

An Example of a System.—Consider the steps in deciding to measure gas exchange at the mouth of a human. The first decision is to exclude all the inanimate objects and all the nonhuman biologic forms from the intended observation. As a second decision, one decides to examine the gas exchange system of the human body and, more specifically, the events that occur at the boundary of the system—that part of the gas exchange system that crosses from the human to the immediate surrounding ambient gas space (the environment). The observer recognizes that there are rules governing the physical properties of the gas, and (he already knows or seeks) the rules that govern the biologic exchange of gas between the atmosphere and the lung. What have been described here are the boundaries of the system and the recognition that a set of laws governs the system.

Limitations in the Application of Instruments

One of the problems in measuring the signal (behavior, response, or output) of a system and attempting to predict what rules or laws govern the system is the changes of the signal that could occur due to the measurement process. There are two ways that the application of instruments can alter the signal to be measured: (1) the instruments may introduce error into the measurement (which is discussed at length in chapter 3), or (2) the instruments may alter the biologic behavior of the tissue, organ, animal, or human under study (which is the subject for discussion here). Sometimes it is not possible to distinguish between these two effects. This is a subtle and problematic area, to which few observers pay much heed.

Kelvin's Rule of Measurement.—Lord Kelvin (the 19th-century physicist) stated that "Measuring instruments must not alter the event being measured." Biologic systems are fragile and responsive, and instruments are cumbersome and intrusive. Therefore, there is a collision between not altering the behavior under study, and yet actually acquiring information about the behavior. A number of factors have been recognized as important in actually or potentially violating this separation of signal from measurement.

Limitation of Response When an Instrument Is Applied.—Consider the universe of behavior of a biologic organism and how it might be restricted by a measuring instrument. If it is necessary to insert a catheter to measure pressure, or if it is necessary to use a mouthpiece to measure gas exchange, then motion of the subject may be limited and this restriction limits the possible range of behavior that could be studied. Although the signal observed might be true and consistent (see chapter 3), it may not be representative of all or most of the behavior of the organism. Furthermore, some biologic signals show changes or development over a longer period of time than the limit of instrument application; conversely, some biologic signals change quicker than some instruments can respond. Therefore, important information may be missed, while the information amassed by the application of instruments may be incorrectly assessed as representative of the entire behavior of the organism. In some measurement schemes, it may be possible to arrange for ambulatory and long-term monitoring instruments, or rapidly responding instruments to avoid this problem. For example, Holter developed electrocardiographic telemetry to observe ambulatory signals.

Alteration of Response When an Instrument Is Applied.—Consider an instrument that is invasive—actually has to pierce the tissue or organ under study. Will the stimulus of attaching the instrument be detected by the system, and will it alter its function? For example, arterial pressure can be measured by direct puncture of the arterial system. The placement of a catheter may provoke pain or anxiety, and possibly alter neurohumoral tone and vascular tone; the catheter itself might alter local vascular endothelium and its behavior and response to stimuli. In an extreme example of careless investigation, severe blood loss could accompany the application of such instrumentation that would obviate the value of the measurement (unless the intent of the investigation was to check the effects of hemorrhage!).

There are other, more subtle examples of this phenomenon. Putting in a mouthpiece for the purpose of measuring gas exchange increases the rate of respiration in humans. In vitro studies on small amounts of tissue and on subcellular processes are especially subject to ambient conditions imposed by experimental design. If this is recognized, an investigator will go to extremes of preparation in order to achieve stable conditions that are thought to be representative of normally occurring—or potentially interesting—conditions.

Classification of Instrumentation

Instrumentation involves the concepts of observation, communication, and control. Based on these concepts, instruments are classified as measurement aids, communication devices, and regulating and following devices (Table 4–1).

Concepts
Observation.—An instrument is used to observe or extend the range of observation of the quantity and quality of a signal.

TABLE 4–1.

Classification of Instrumentation

CONCEPT	APPLICATION
Observation	Measurement aids (most instruments)
Communication	Communication devices (display devices, recorders, cables, telemetry links)
Regulation	Regulating and following devices (servomechanisms and therapeutic devices)

Communication.—Instruments communicate these observations between themselves, other devices used in measurement, and ultimately to the human in a form that is interpretable and usable.

Regulation.—Instruments can be used to control the flow and utilization of information, and to regulate the system under study.

Application of Concepts

Measurement Aides.—These devices are used to *observe* a signal that is beyond the ability of the human to observe either because of quantitative and/or qualitative limitations of the senses, or because it is necessary to extend the senses of the human to observe the signal more completely or accurately. Most of what we think of as instruments fall into this category. For example, an electrode and high gain electrical amplifier are measurement aides that allow us to observe what our senses are not capable of detecting—cardiac electrical activity. A pneumotachygraph head, differential pressure transducer, and amplifier allow the quantitative measurement of ventilation, which is an improvement over the detection of respiration by observation of condensate on a mirror by a detective in a murder novel.

Communication Devices.—These devices *communicate* information between instruments or, after translation to a form that can be understood by human intelligence, between instruments and people. Many of these devices lead relatively unrecognized lives in the form of cables, signal transmission devices, and telemetry links. They do become highly visible at the end of the instrumentation chain in the form of recording and display instruments.

Regulating and Following Devices (Servomechanisms).—These are two-stage devices that first *observe* the signal and then *emit* a signal that is either constant (regulating device) or variable in order to restore the observed signal to a set point (following device). The signal we would expect to be emitted from an instrument that was connected to a human would probably control a device used for therapy or treatment. Because of the complexity of biologic systems, and the well-founded discomfort that an instrument could fail or be inappropriately applied, there are relatively few of these servomechanism instruments that are applicable as therapeutic devices to humans.

An electronic cardiac pacemaker is perhaps an excellent example of a therapeutic *regulating* instrument. The first stage of this device observes the spontaneous heart rate. When the heart rate is lower than a predetermined rate, the second stage of the pacemaker discharges an electrical energy pulse in order to stimulate the myocardium and initiate a cardiac action potential. However, many versions of the pacemaker have no ability to observe whether this discharge is successful in actually capturing the heart and stimulating an action potential. Therefore, we can classify it as a regulating device, but not a *servomechanism*.

A newer generation of pacemakers has some desirable properties that suggest that they are servomechanisms. These pacemakers actually detect whether there has been a successful capture of the heart rhythm, and they can adjust energy output if capture requirements change. As another example, the glucose clamp is a servomechanism instrument that is capable of controlling the infusions of glucose and insulin intravenously into a human in response to the continuous measurement of blood glucose so as to achieve a predetermined level of blood glucose. However, this device has not yet been adapted for long-term and widespread therapeutic use.

Although servomechanisms that provide therapy or treatment to a biologic system are infrequent, they are used ubiquitously as components to improve the function of instruments.

The Chain of Instrumentation

Conceptually and practically, an instrument can perform only a single function. However, it is almost always necessary to perform multiple operations on a biologic signal before it can be measured. Therefore, multiple instruments are arranged as a series or series-parallel chain that is suitable for this process (Fig 4–1). Because many in-

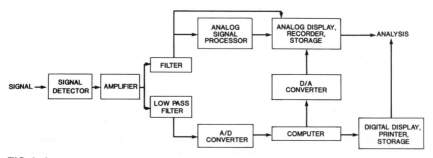

FIG 4–1.
The chain of instrumentation. Instruments perform a single function. In order to measure a biologic signal, it is necessary to assemble instruments in a series and series-parallel arrangement. The figure suggests one such arrangement that includes analog and digital instruments.

struments are packages or combinations of individual instruments, it is easy to forget that applied instrumentation is a series of steps. Because of this bundling, which is analogous to a "combination" drug, it is possible to use or purchase an incorrect instrument if one or more of the bundled instruments has a specification that is not correct for the signal to be observed, or the process to be regulated.

In the chapters to follow, we will discuss how instruments convert biologic signals into a form that can be detected, conditioned, displayed, archived, and eventually analyzed by the observer. The instruments described in chapters 5, 6, and 7 are considered *analog* instruments because they treat the information content as *continuous*. In chapter 8, we will discuss *digital* instruments (computers) that treat the information content of the signal in a noncontinuous or *discrete* form.

Signal Detectors (Chaper 5)

The mass and energy forms of most biologic phenomena mentioned in chapter 2 cannot readily be measured or quantified by the five human senses. Therefore, it is necessary to use a device that specifically detects a biologic signal and converts it to one that is more suitable for measurement by an instrument. These devices are called *signal detectors*. Electrodes and transducers are examples of this class of instruments.

Signal Conditioners (Chapter 6)

Signal conditioners operate on the transduced signal and prepare it for display and recording.

Amplifiers.—An amplifier is an instrument that alters the energy (usually increases the energy) of a signal without changing the information contained in the signal. This amplification of signal energy is necessary because the magnitude of the energy of most biologic signals is small, and because the energy output of the earlier instruments of the instrumentation chain—such as signal detectors and preamplifiers—is not usually large enough for measurement purposes. Two benefits derive from amplification. First, when a signal is amplified its level can be more precisely resolved. This type of amplifier is inserted immediately after a signal detector and is called an *instrumentation amplifier*. Second, when a signal is amplified its energy level becomes sufficient for the operation of other instruments in the instrumentation chain that require a high power signal, such as a recorder. This type of amplifier is used at multiple points in the instrumentation chain and is called a *driver* or *power amplifier*.

Filters.—A filter is an instrument that selectively removes or limits part of the bandwidth of the signal. High-pass filters (filters that remove low-frequency components of the signal), low-pass filters (filters that remove high-frequency components of the signal), and bandpass filters (filters that remove both high- and low-frequency components of the signal) are especially important to remove extraneous or unwanted parts of the frequency content of a signal.

Signal Processors.—A signal processor is an instrument that operates on a signal by either a mathematical or logical operation. The object of a signal processor is to assist in the analysis of a signal, usually by extracting some important part of the signal or by performing a mathematical or logical process on the signal, such as the four basic mathematical functions or more complex algebraic ones.

Display Devices and Recorders (Chapter 7)
In order for a human to observe the transduced and conditioned signal, it is necessary that some sensory display (usually visual) be made of the signal and, frequently, that some permanent record be made for purposes of review, analysis, and possibly further signal processing. There is a wide variety of media and instruments on which this recording can be done. This includes electromagnetic media (such as magnetic tape), photographic media, and paper media (such as strip chart recordings made with ink).

Cables and Connectors (Chapter 7)

The individual components and instruments of the instrument chain are held together and transmit information by links—the connecting wires, connecting ports (connectors), and communication devices. They have a critical role in error-free transmission of the information within the chain.

Computers (Chapter 8)

Although we've all become accustomed to the prodigious calculating, data storage, and data retrieval capabilities of computers, they are also capable of serving very successfully as surrogate digital instruments in place of analog ones. All of the instrument functions mentioned above (transduction is still in dispute) can be performed by a computer.

The Instrumentation Chain:
I. Signal Detectors

In this chapter, we will explore devices used to detect biologic signals—electrodes and transducers. *A signal detector converts the mass or energy form of the original signal to another form—almost always an electrical form.* As an example of signal detectors, we'll pick up the thread of analogy about music signals that we laid down in chapter 2. There, we characterized the signal properties of music as a model for biologic signals. Here we'll discuss instruments that are used to observe music signals, which are colloquially called a component stereo system. I will use this system over the next few chapters as an example of an instrumentation chain.

The stereo system is used with a variety of music signal inputs. The signal inputs may come from a microphone, from a radio, from a tape player, from a phonograph, or from a compact disc. Each of these devices has a signal detector: the microphone has a crystal or magnetic element; the radio has a tuner; the tape player has a head; the phonograph turntable has a cartridge or needle; and the compact disc has a laser. The object of each of these devices is to detect the information in the music signal and convert it to a form the stereo instrument can use. The crystal or magnetic element in the microphone converts sound energy (vibrations) into electrical energy. The tuner in the radio converts electromagnetic radiation into electrical energy. The head of a tape player converts a magnetic field into electrical energy. The cartridge of a phonograph converts a mechanical displacement of the needle as it tracks the pits and grooves of a phonograph record into electrical energy. The laser of a compact disc player does the same.

Biologic signal detectors do the same thing: they take some characteristic or property of the biologic signal and translate it into a form—usually electrical energy—that is usable by the instruments.

WHAT YOU NEED TO KNOW

1. *Signal detectors,* including electrodes and transducers, receive as an input a biologic signal in its original mass or energy form, convert that signal into a different form without altering the information content of the original signal, and provide an output that is usable by another instrument.

2. *Electrodes* are interface devices that couple bioelectricity to galvanic electricity, or are used to generate or detect an electromagnetic field.

3. *Strain guage transducers* convert a deformation of a material due to pressure, force or length into an alteration of an electrical property. In turn, the electrical property is converted by a bridge circuit to electrical energy.

4. *Piezoelectric crystals* convert deformation due to pressure, motion, sound, or other mechanical forces to electrical energy. Conversely, crystals may be subjected to electrical energy in order to produce a mechanical deformation and sound waves.

5. *Thermistors* and *thermocouples* convert temperature to resistance and electrical energy, respectively. The electrical energy produced by a thermocouple is used directly without further modification. The resistance change of a thermistor may be converted through a bridge circuit to electrical energy.

6. *Photoelectric* and *scintigraphic detectors* convert electromagnetic energy to changes of electrical properties or light energy, respectively. Altered electrical properties from a photoelectric detector may

be converted through a bridge circuit to electrical energy. Light energy from a scintigraphic detector may be converted through a photoelectric detector and then a bridge circuit to electrical energy.

Principles of Signal Detection

Signal detectors are the Rosetta stone of instruments: they take indecipherable biologic signals and make that information "understandable" to other instruments in the instrumentation chain. Signal detectors perform this function by converting the mass or energy of the biologic signal into another energy form—usually electrical—and by making that energy available as the input to another instrument.

Why Have Signal Detectors?

Biologic signals are really not suitable for direct connection to most of the instrumentation chain. The first stumbling block to their measurement is that their signal form is not suitable for processing by electronic instrumentation. The major function of a signal detector is to convert faithfully the information content of the biologic signal to a form that is suitable for use by the remainder of the instrumentation chain. For electronic instruments, the required form is that of electrical energy.

Transducible Property

The key that permits the detection of a signal in a biologic system is called the *transducible property* of the system. It is that characteristic of the signal that allows a physical device to detect the signal and thereby to infer the function or structure of the system under study. In the example cited previously, the sound vibrations associated with music are the transducible property when a microphone is used. The other transducible properties of music cited above (electromagnetic radiation, magnetic field, pits on a smooth surface) are also the transducible property of music; they were all purposefully designed to take advantage of special signal detectors.

In biologic systems it's important to identify the transducible property of the system. Historically, many investigations of biologic systems were shaped by what signal detectors were available, and by what transducible property was recognized. Sometimes, when an important transducible property was recognized, signal detectors evolved over a long period to detect that property. This has happened with the instrumentation used to measure blood flow in the cardiovascular system. Sometimes, the availability of a signal detector finally coaxed investigators into searching for a transducible property. This has happened with imaging tools such as ultrasound, digital x-ray, nuclear scintigraphy, and nuclear magnetic resonance where the signal detectors were widely used outside of biology before their application to biology.

Ideal Properties of Signal Detectors

There are a number of characteristics that should ideally characterize the properties of a signal detector.

Specificity.—The accurate and precise measurement of a biologic signal importantly depends on the ability of the signal detector to detect only one form or, especially, one subtype of signal and to distinguish it from other biological signals and extraneous signals. This is called *specificity*. Within each biologic system or tissue, there may be more than one signal emitted as the behavior of that system. In the cardiovascular system the choices are among bioelectricity, pressure, flow, motion, and biochemistry. Ideally, a signal detector should discriminate among these.

Of equal importance, and more problematic, is the discrimination of similar signals between biologic systems or tissues. For example, bioelectricity is generated by a plethora of biologic systems. Measurement of brain, nerve, or muscle bioelectrical phenomena are frequently overwhelmed or distorted by the presence of cardiac electrical activity. Ideally, a signal detector would be specific for each of these.

Applicability.—It should be possible to actually use the conceptual design and physical package that constitutes the signal detector in the measurement of biologic signals; this is called *applicability*. A signal detector usually has to be physically close to, and frequently in contact with, the source of the signal. Many otherwise excellent concepts and physical designs of transducers are not applicable because they encumber the signal source. Even when such problems are present, such signal detectors are sometimes used with the acknowledgment that they may limit or alter biologic behavior. For example, ultrasound crystals, when attached to an arterial wall for the purpose of measuring changes in diameter of the artery, mechanically load and restrict wall motion.

Errors.—A signal detector should cause minimum error. We reviewed the types of error that instruments can make in chapter 3, and all of these are possible with respect to signal detectors. Congruent with all instruments, transducers must have amplitude linearity and a bandwidth adequate for the intended purpose. We have previously described the measurement of amplitude linearity in simplest terms of the maximum deviation from linearity of output vs. input, as well as the more sophisticated term of total harmonic distortion. This deviation should be kept quite small, perhaps no more than 1% within the intended range of operation of the signal detector. The bandwidth of the transducer should be adequate for the intended use. This depends on the frequency spectrum of the signal and on the information to be derived from the signal.

Design Characteristics

There are a number of characteristics that describe the operation of signal detectors.

Energy Requirements.—Signal detectors are classified as either active or passive devices, depending on whether they require an external source of energy in order to function. As confusing as it may sound, an active signal detector requires an external source of energy in order to produce an electrical output, whereas a passive transducer does not. The external energy required in an active signal detector is frequently used to power a Wheatstone bridge.

Wheatstone Bridge.—The Wheatstone bridge is a very useful and simple electrical circuit that is used for the precision measurement of small changes of electrical voltage in the circuit. Why is such a circuit of value in a transducer?

The sensing elements of transducers, which are commonly resistances, or resistance-like devices such as reactances (capacitors and inductors), change their level of resistance in response to a signal. Sometimes, the change of resistance is quite large and changes of resistance can be satisfactorily resolved by a simple circuit. However, frequently the change of resistance is only a few percent. It is very important, but at the same time very difficult, to be able to measure this change in resistance precisely. The series-parallel arrangement of the resistors in the Wheatstone bridge circuit is governed by a circuit theory of flow of current, which causes a precision change of voltage in the circuit in proportion to a small change in resistance. One or more of the resistors (the "arms" of the bridge) is the actual element involved in signal detection. It changes its resistance in response to the signal, which causes a precise change in voltage output of the bridge.

When a resistor is used as the sensing element of the bridge circuit, excitation (external energy) to the bridge may be supplied by a DC or AC power source. Changes of resistance in response to the signal alter the distribution of current flow within the bridge and therefore alter voltage measured at the output of the bridge. When reactances, such as inductors and capacitors, are used as the sensing elements of the bridge circuit, excitation to the bridge is supplied by an AC power source. Changes of reactance in response to the signal alter the distribution of AC current flow within the bridge and therefore alter AC voltage measured at the output of the bridge.

Stages.—Signal detectors may have one or more stages to their function. Sometimes signal detectors are single-stage devices and transduce the biologic signal directly into the desired form. Electrodes are an example of this. They transduce ionic electricity of the excitable tissue into galvanic electricity that is suitable for other instruments to use. Sometimes, signal detectors are multistage devices so that they can achieve an appropriate output. For example, respiratory flow can be detected by a pneumotachygraph transducer, which converts flow to a pressure differential; this pressure differential is detected by a pressure transducer and subsequently converted to an electrical output. As another example, cardiac motion may be detected by the spatial position of a radioisotope within the heart, and then the ionizing radiation produced by the decay of this radioisotope is detected by a scintillation crystal and converted to an electrical output.

Electrodes

Electrodes are useful for the measurement of at least four different types of biologic events: spontaneous electrical activity, in which the electrodes are used to sense the phenomenon; stimulated electrical activity, in which the electrodes are used to transmit the electrical stimulation to excitable tissue; motion, volume, and flow events, in which the electric field generated by the electrodes is distorted by the mass event to be detected; and ionic concentrations, in which the amount of a chemical compound is measured.

Theory

Bioelectrical events are ionic phenomena. They occur because a potential difference is generated whenever different concentrations of the same conductor are separated by a semipermeable membrane. In the cell, Na^+ and K^+ solutions of different concentrations exist across the semipermeable cell membrane. The potential difference across the membrane is in the order of a few dozen microvolts. The potential generated by a whole organ such as the heart may be a few millivolts.

A potential difference is also generated whenever a conductor comes into contact with an electrolyte. This is called the electrical half-cell potential. Ions from the conductor attempt to enter the electrolyte and ions from the electrolyte attempt to enter the conductor. Electrodes convert this ionic potential difference into a galvanic potential difference, that is, one that is useful for transmission to another instrument. When used as electrodes, the ionic electricity of the biologic signal source is transmitted through an electrolyte to a metal electrode. The source of the electrolyte may be the fluid around the tissue which is the source of the bioelectricity; or, it may be an artificial electrolyte placed between the source of the signal and the electrode (electrode jelly).

Application

Electrodes have certain important properties that govern their suitability as signal detectors. Because they are the proximate element in the instrumentation chain, and usually touch or surround the signal source, they must not interfere with the production of the biologic event (see chapter 4), unless they are stimulating electrodes. If applied directly to the subject or organ under study, they must be nontoxic and they must be applicable to the locus of generation of the biologic event. In addition to these physical properties, electrodes have been discovered to have a complex series of electrical properties that govern their utility. There is a wide variety of electrode types based on material of construction and configuration, each constructed for a specific purpose (Fig 5–1).

Drift and Offset.—Because electrodes are conductors, they develop a half-cell potential when they contact an ionic solution. This battery-like potential is in addition to and, from the signal detection standpoint, irrelevant to measurement of the biologic electrical event. However, this electrode voltage offset is transmitted to the next instrument, the amplifier. If it were constant, the electrode offset potential could be removed or cancelled out by the amplifier offset capabilities (see chapter 6). Unfortunately, it is not, and so some other mechanism must be found to eliminate or minimize offset potential. These time-dependent variations are called *drift* when they are slowly occurring phenomena, and *noise* when they are rapidly occurring. Drift may be

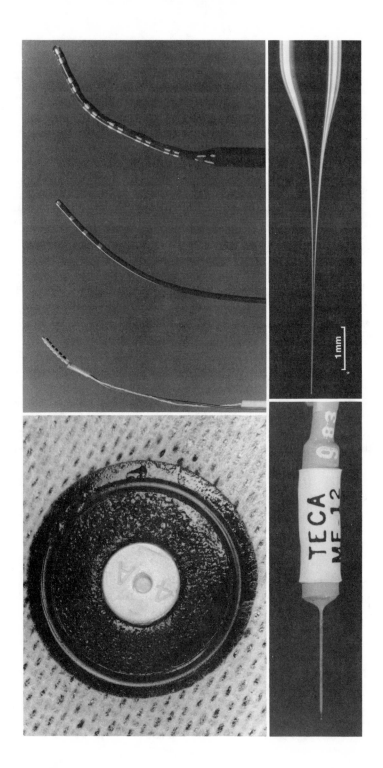

handled by using AC coupling or high-pass filtering, and noise may be handled by low-pass filtering. Both are discussed in the amplifier section of chapter 6.

Construction.—Surface and tissue electrodes are usually made of solid materials. A wide variety of metals are good conductors and have a large half-cell potential, which make them candidates as electrodes. Drift and noise are reduced by using pure metals (e.g., >99.99% pure silver), and by adding a thin layer of the salt of the metal on the surface of the electrode. The most favorable example of this construction technique is the silver/silver chloride electrode.

Microelectrodes, or electrodes that are small enough to contact the cell membrane surface or puncture and enter an individual cell, may be made of very fine electrode wire or, more commonly, electrolyte solutions contained within a glass micropipette.

Electrodes behave as if they are small batteries or capacitors that hold and maintain a small voltage or charge until linked to an amplifier. Electrode pairs or groups must be made of the same material and connected through the same electrolyte to the biologic object in order to reduce the effects that two different battery poles can have on amplification and recording instruments. Over the first few seconds after connection, a definite discharge takes place that may alter the signal properties or the signal stability as observed on the recording instrument. Therefore, it is always advisable to wait a few minutes after electrode connection before initiating signal measurement. This signal distortion will also be a function of the filtering properties of the amplifier.

A further problem with electrodes occurs because electrodes are

---

FIG 5–1.
Electrodes. These are a few examples of the materials and configurations of electrodes. *(Bottom left)* typical skin electrode for measurement of human ECG. This electrode (silver/silver chloride) is a solid 8.5-mm disc mounted in the center of an adhesive pad, and covered with a pad that contains electrolyte (that pad has been removed for clearer viewing of the electrode). *(Top left)* typical catheter-mounted electrode used in the measurement of local cardiac electrical activity. The electrodes *(platinum rings)* are mounted as a series near the catheter tip. For surface measurements of electrical activity, the catheter on the left is placed on the surface of the heart. For intravascular measurements of electrical activity, the two catheters on the right are passed intravascularly to sites of interest on the subendocardium of the heart. *(Bottom right)* typical plunge electrode used in the measurement of neural activity, or other electrical activity. The 10-mm long platinum electrode needle pierces the skin or tissue under study and overlays or lays within the site of activity. *(Top right)* typical microelectrode used in the measurement of intracellular electrical activity. The tip of the glass capillary (a few microns in diameter) punctures the cell membrane. The capillary is fllled with an electrolyte, usually KCl.

used in pairs to record potential differences between two sites, and because the two electrodes may exhibit small differences in resistance (actually impedance). This resistance imbalance, in association with the small current flow through the electrodes, can induce an offset or drift error. This can be minimized by electrodes that contact a large surface area, and the use of electrolyte materials and equal connecting wire lengths. In extreme circumstances, impedance can be measured in each electrode arm, and efforts expended to adjust for equality. Electrode usage still remains an art with slowly appreciated principles and practical advancements.

Electrodes for Spontaneous Electrical Signals

These devices are used to transmit a spontaneous action potential from individual cells or from whole organs such as from the brain, nerves, muscles, heart, gut, or specialized electrical organ. These events are ionic, and therefore are not suitable for direct electrical recording. Hence, the function of the electrode is to "transduce" these ionic events into electrical events. Typically, the level of voltage potential of an individual cell is in the microvolt range, whereas that of an organ is in the millivolt range.

Surface Electrodes.—Electrodes may lie on the surface of the source of the bioelectrical signal. It is frequently unsatisfactory to attempt to make continuous direct contact with the surface to which the electrodes are attached. Because a flat metal electrode will not make a secure and constant contact with the skin, good contact is maintained through an ionic medium of a mild electrolyte jelly. Because of the high input impedence of subsequent amplifiers (chapter 6) almost any weak electrolyte will do just fine. For example, moist alcohol wipes, which are readily available in patient care areas, can be used for very short-term clinical purposes. These conductive media ensure that surface imperfections and small movements of the surface will still allow continuous contact with the electrode. To encourage the coupling through the skin surface, it is necessary to abrade the poorly conducting horny skin layer, which has poor electrical conducting properties, and to expose the more fluid and ionic-rich dermal layers. Thus, vigorous rubbing or actual light sanding of the skin is in order.

Plunge Electrodes.—Electrodes may penetrate the surface of the source of the bioelectricity. These electrodes make direct contact with the tissue under study or with the ionic milieu of the skin. For purpose of strength, they may be constructed of stainless steel, but will frequently be platinum coated. These wires may be inserted directly into the tissue or through the hollow core of a larger and stronger needle that has punctured the surface of the organ to be studied. In addition to the comments on offset and drift caused by charge on contact electrodes, plunge electrodes may accumulate biologic materials of different resistance properties on their surface, which may cause further instability of signal level.

Electrodes for Stimulation and Generation of an Electrical Field

These electrodes are energized by an external power supply and either stimulate an excitable tissue in order to observe its response (electrical, mechanical, or otherwise) or generate an electrical field that will be distorted by the motion of some or part of the organism within the field.

Stimulating Electrodes.—These are used widely in studies of the brain, nerves, muscle, or heart, for two purposes. One purpose is to substitute stimulated behavior for the normally limited range of electrical activity of that organ in order to observe more fully all of its possible behavior. Regional excitation of heart or brain may yield valuable localized or general behavior that would not be apparent from spontaneously generated electrical activity.

The second purpose for which stimulating electrodes are used is to remove the uncertainty and nonspontaneity of organ electrical events. It may be desired to study the effects of a spontaneous but infrequent electrical event. The choices are either to monitor and be prepared to record that event continuously, or to stimulate the onset of that event to remove the unpredictable element of spontaneity. For the stimulating electrode, an extremely important assumption that must be made is that the event that has been stimulated is part of the spectrum of events of which that organ is possible, and/or that the information derived from that stimulation is biologically relevant.

Impedance Electrodes.—Impedance electrodes are also widely used to study biologic events. The electrodes are used to generate an electrical field that surrounds the signal source and to detect signal by observing its distortion of the electrical field. In this way it is possible to observe electrical events, motion events including translational and rotational activity, and mass transfer events including the flow of conductive materials such as blood. Because of the noninvasive capabilities of impedance electrodes, they have been tried for a wide variety of signals. Their utility is greatly limited by lack of specificity and difficulty in calibration. Therefore, their greatest use is in the detection of qualitative events. However, current interest in their noninvasive application is maintained in the detection of respiratory events and cardiac output. When invasively applied to a device that encircles an organ or enters a hollow organ, precise and accurate measurement of volume and motion has been demonstrated.

Impedance electrodes are applied usually in the form of an impedance bridge—that is, two or more electrodes are used as variable resistors, and current is passed through the electrodes (see below for a further discussion of bridges). The type of excitation applied is high-frequency AC. Both the pain perception and the tissue response to AC stimulation at any given current level are highly dependent on the frequency of stimulation. When extremely high rates of stimulation occur, usually far in excess of 10,000 Hz (cycles per second), excitable tissue stimulation does *not* take place and therefore the danger of harmful excitation (e.g., ventricular fibrillation) is avoided. However, electrical energy still enters the body or organ encircled or girdled by the impedance electrodes. Under those circumstances, the electrical energy is dissipated as heat energy. Small amounts or short periods of electrical energy delivered at high frequency will be harmlessly dissipated. Larger amounts or longer periods of high-frequency stimulation can have biologic effects of local heating of tissue. These may be detrimental, as in thermal destruction, or therapeutically beneficial, as in diathermy.

Biochemical Electrodes

These electrodes are used to measure concentrations of molecules. Some are used to measure ions and others are used to measure nonionic molecules. Their membranes have to exhibit a high degree of selectivity for the molecular species because the biologic milieu is teeming with multiple molecular signals. They are extremely popular because of their simplicity (compared to alternative chemical procedures), precision, low cost, and direct connection to other instrumentation. Electrodes are available that directly measure the concentrations of oxygen, carbon dioxide, and pH by producing a current flow in proportion to concentration. They are useful for measuring oxygen and carbon dioxide in both the gaseous and fluid phases. Carbon dioxide in blood can also be measured by observation of changes in pH in response to adding calibrated concentrations of carbon dioxide because of the known relationship of the acid-base bicarbonate buffer system. Electrodes are also available for monovalent and divalent ionic species, glucose, lactate, and pyruvate. The size and chemical instability of the electrodes limit their application during in vivo measurements; for continuous on-line measurement, the electrodes may be adapted to extracorporeal sampling cuvette, and the fluid may be returned to the organism if needed. There are known limitations with respect to drift of the calibration, aging (which causes a deterioration of signal output), and time response (which may be on the order of seconds).

Strain Gauge Transducers

A strain gauge transducer is a signal detector that is used to measure the physical properties of force and pressure.

How a Strain Gauge Works

Theory.—The principle of the strain gauge is a deformation (strain, or change of length per unit length) of the sensing component of the transducer in response to mechanical change applied to the transducer. If the transducer is attached to an object that generates force, such as a strip of muscle, then the deformation can be expressed as a force measurement in units of grams and dynes. If the transducer is pressurized by a liquid (including air or gas), such as blood in a cavity of an organ or saline in a catheter placed in a blood vessel, and the area of the sensing element is known, then the deformation can be expressed as a pressure measurement in units of dynes/cm^2 or mm Hg.

Construction.—A number of ingenious ways have been proposed and used to measure the deformation of the sensing element of a strain gauge, and thereby the force or pressure of the signal. Current techniques have largely focused on the ability of certain materials to change their electrical characteristics in response to deformation. For these materials, the larger the deformation, the greater the change of resistance, capacitance, inductance, or reluctance (the magnetic equivalent of resistance).

Unlike the galvanic electrical output of electrodes, these changes in electrical characteristics of the strain gauge transducer do not directly produce an electrical output; that is, changes of resistance, reactance, and magnetic field do not produce an electrical signal that can be passed to another instrument. Therefore, some device is required to convert these changes in resistance, reactance, and magnetic field to an electrical output. This device is a Wheatstone bridge for transducers that use resistors and reactances (chapter 4), or a transformer for transducers that use a magnetic core. The transducer accurately and precisely changes its voltage output in proportion to changes of the

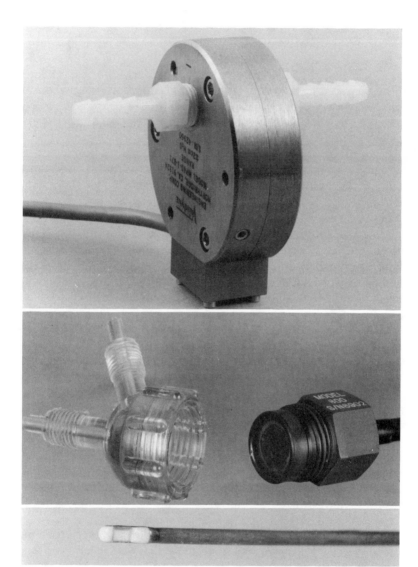

FIG 5–2.
Pressure transducers. A few examples of the configurations of pressure transducers. *(Top)* typical differential pressure transducer used in conjunction with a pneumotachygraph head for measurement of respiratory flow. There is a pressure port on each side of the sensing diaphragm. The deformation of the diaphragm, and therefore change of electrical characteristics, is proportional to the pressure differential. *(Center)* typical fluid-filled pressure transducer (manometer) used in conjunction with an intravascular catheter. The clear plastic dome *(left)* seals fluid against the sensor diaphragm and allows the connection of a

sensing element. The strain gauge is an active transducer, which requires a power source or *excitation*. The voltage output of the bridge can be amplified and recorded as the signal of interest.

Types and Application

Strain gauge transducers have been produced in a wide variety of shapes and forms (Fig 5–2). The materials or components that act as sensing elements are usually bonded to a diaphragm to provide a known and constant surface area of exposure to the signal, and to protect the biologic source from the sensor and the sensor from the biologic source.

Connection to Signal Source Through a Catheter.—In the most widely used form of strain gauge transducer, a dome containing liquid or gas is placed over a diaphragm that contains the sensing element or active arm of the bridge. The dome is then attached through a fluid- or gas-filled tube or connector to the site of pressure or force.

The advantages of this construction are that it leaves the transducer external to the source of pressure or force signal and allows the transducer to be observed, tended to, and calibrated during measurement. It also protects the transducer from possible harm at the site of signal generation. Even if failure of operation of the strain gauge occurs, as a worst-case scenario, the transducer can be replaced without grossly interrupting the course of the measurement. The disadvantage is that indirect connection of the sensing element always leaves open the question of whether or not what is observed by the sensing element is truly the signal generated at its source. A gross example of this is a kink—obstruction or loss of continuity in the connecting apparatus between the transducer and the signal source. A more subtle but pervasive problem is the alteration (usually degradation) of frequency response that occurs as a result of the connecting apparatus.

Direct Contact With Signal Source.—In response to these problems with indirect connection of the signal with the transducer, it has

---

fluid-filled catheter to the transducer. The cable from the transducer *(right)* contains a hollow tube that is open to the ambient pressure and that provides a reference pressure for the sensor. *(Bottom)* typical catheter-tipped pressure transducer (manometer) used for the measurement of intravascular pressure. This is miniaturized version of the fluid-filled transducer, but mounted on a catheter. The catheter is passed to the site of measurement from within the vascular tree and is directly contacted by the source of pressure. However, the principle of operation is the same as the fluid-filled manometer.

been desirable to place the sensing element of the transducer in direct contact with the signal source. The transducer can be fabricated onto a catheter so that it can be passed from a remote site to the site of interest; or it can be fabricated as a sensing element alone that is surgically implanted at the site of interest.

The advantages of this design are that one has increased confidence that the observed signal and the true signal are the same. Frequency response may be an order of magnitude ($\times 10$) better. However, there are a number of disadvantages. Biologic systems are relatively small in scale and fragile. Until recently, the sensing element has not been small enough to allow direct contact, or durable enough to tolerate the forces that are generated during passage to the site of interest or that are present during use while in place. Particularly vexing is the inability under many circumstances to calibrate the transducer *in situ* or readily replace it should it fail during the actual time of signal measurement.

Specifications

Sensitivity or Gain.—As described previously, the three quantities that characterize the operation of a strain gauge transducer are the signal input, the voltage output of the strain gauge in response to the signal, and the voltage mode and quantity of excitation of the gauge. These three are expressed together as the *sensitivity or gain* of the gauge.

The form of the relationship among these three quantities is

"x" microvolts output/mm Hg signal input/volt of bridge excitation.

(The units of dimensions of pressure could be different, e.g., cm H_2O or pounds per square inch). It is an unusual form of expressing gain because it includes not only the customary ratio of output to input, but also includes the effect of voltage excitation on the gain of the device. The higher the sensitivity or gain, the greater is the electrical output for any level of signal input at a particular level of excitation. It is desirable to have a strain gauge with a high sensitivity because of increased resolution of the signal.

Reference Pressure.—My mechanical engineering dynamics teacher, on the first day of class, held a board eraser stationary in front of the blackboard and asked, "What's the speed of this eraser?" The correct answer is first to query, "In relationship to what other object?" In relationship to the blackboard, 0; in relationship to someone walking by in the corridor outside the classroom, a few miles per hour; in relationship to the position of the sun, about 70,000 miles per hour. That is, all physical levels of measurement are relative or in reference to some other level.

The same is true for pressure. Pressure transducers measure a pressure level in reference to another pressure level. Although the user is frequently unaware of this reference pressure, its importance cannot be overemphasized because all transducers require a calibration in relation to the reference pressure. The reference level is determined by what pressure exists on the side of the diaphragm where the strain sensing element is located. Three types of pressure may be used: absolute zero, atmospheric, and differential.

Absolute zero may be used as the reference pressure when the transducer and its connecting and supporting cables will be inaccessible during use and there will be no opportunity to calibrate in reference to a pressure. The level of pressure that is measured is relative to absolute zero. Wholly implantable transducers may be evacuated and sealed on the sensing side of the diaphragm. These are used to monitor pressure in cavities, vascular spaces, and solid tissues.

Atmospheric pressure may be used as the reference pressure when the sensing side of the diaphragm can be open to ambient pressure. This is usually accomplished by placing a narrow-gauge air-filled tube within the electrical cable that leads to the transducer. The tube is open at the side of the sensing element, and open to atmosphere at the other end of the cable. Most external and catheter-tipped transducers are constructed in this manner. Some care has to be exercised to avoid crimping or plugging this tube because the reference will become uncertain. Atmospheric pressure is about 760 mm Hg higher than absolute zero, but varies according to height above sea level and weather conditions.

Differential pressure is used when the intent is to measure the relative or difference in pressure across the diaphragm of the transducer. In use, each side of the diapraghm is connected to a site of pressure, and the difference between the two sides is measured. Differential pressure transducers are used to measure the difference in pressure between two anatomical sites, such as the difference between the esophageal pressure (presumed pleural) and the stomach pressure. They are also used to measure differential pressure across a device that is itself acting as a signal detector, such as a pneumotachygraph head which converts airflow to a differential pressure.

Range.—Pressure and force transducers operate within a range of signal input and voltage excitation. The range of signal input is limited by the ability of these transducers to undergo deformation without rupturing or permanently distorting the diaphragm and the sensing element. Fragility and range are two severe limitations in the operation of this type of transducer.

An instrument manufacturer will frequently have a line of transducers that operate on the same principle and have the same basic construction, but individual models are optimized for a particular range of pressure. For example, the range of pressure signals generated by a pneumotachygraph head in response to airflow are small (0 to about 1 mm Hg differential); the ranges generated by gastrointestinal pressure are larger (slightly less than zero to a few mm Hg); and the largest are generated by pleural pressure (as much as 20 mm Hg on either side of zero) and by the vascular system (slightly less than zero to a few hundred mm Hg). In each application it is advisable to use a transducer which has been optimized for that range of force or pressure.

Errors.—Because they are mechanical devices, strain gauge transducers are likely to have limitations of amplitude linearity, bandwidth, and frequency response. The latter is especially problematic in strain gauges that are applied through indirect connection, because the properties of the tubing, and the fluid contained within the tubing (including possible contamination by gas), may considerably degrade bandwidth. This is shown for a pressure transducer (chapter 9, Fig 9–3) with different tubing connections and with gas in the tubing. Notice that all the phenomena described in chapter 3, including resonance and attenuation, can be seen with pressure transducers and their connections.

Manufacturers provide data on bandwidth as part of the specifications of the strain gauge transducer. My experience is that the reported values of bandwidth are not always realistic during actual use: sometimes the high-frequency response is not as good as the specifications would suggest. Especially troublesome with fluid-filled transducers that require tubing and catheter connections is the absence of reliable and practical data during "field" conditions—that is, systems during actual use. Even if such were available for each catheter and transducer combination, frequency response is readily altered during application unless there is attention to minute details of connections and gas bubbles. The rules of thumb for these catheters and tubing are that high-frequency response degrades (1) as length increases; (2) as diameter changes outside of a range of values (very large or very small diameters); and (3) as material of construction becomes more pliable.

Piezoelectric Crystals

A piezoelectric crystal is a material that reversibly converts electrical energy to mechanical (pressure, hence *piezo*) deformation.

The original biomedical application of such crystals was the detection and analysis of sound waves originating from such sources as heart sounds and Korotkoff sounds (sounds associated with cuff measurement of blood pressure). The former is still used as a teaching tool to assist novices in the auscultation of the heart. The latter finds widespread application in biomedical instrumentation that is used for the noninvasive measurement of blood pressure.

Piezoelectric crystals have found much broader and sophisticated uses in the past 20 years. One important clinical and basic research application is the noninvasive imaging (echo) of internal organs including the heart, liver, gallbladder, pancreas, kidneys, and uterus (including fetus). Another important basic research application is the invasive measurement of the dynamic dimensions of the heart. Another innovative application in clinical and basic research is the measurement of blood flow velocity within the heart and blood vessels (Doppler).

How a Piezoelectric Crystal Works

Theory.—Certain anisotropic (having different structural properties in different planes of the material) crystals produce a temporary deformation of the shape of the crystal when they are subjected to an electrical charge (piezoelectric effect); or they produce a temporary charge at the surface of the crystal when they are deformed (inverse piezoelectric effect). The naturally occurring materials including quartz, lithium sulfate, and potassium sodium tartrate, and the artificial ceramic materials, including barium titanate and lead zirconate, show strong piezoelectric properties.

When deformed by a force, a voltage equivalent of a fraction of a volt (but a tiny current) is produced. The ratio of charge produced per deforming force is called the *piezoelectric constant*. This can be amplified, signal conditioned, and displayed so as to reveal some information about the characteristics of the deforming force. Conversely, when subjected to an electrical field, a deformation can be produced that will produce a mechanical vibration in the surrounding medium—a sound.

Construction.—Transducers have been fashioned from piezoelectric crystals to take advantage of either or both of the above-mentioned phenomena (Fig 5–3).

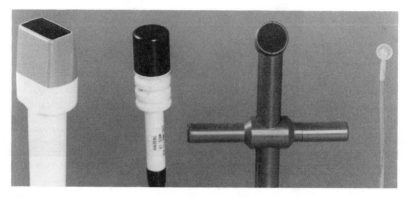

FIG 5–3.
Piezoelectric crystals. A few examples of the different configurations and applications of such crystals. *(Left)* a combination echo and Doppler crystal used for cardiac and vascular imaging. This transducer is applied at the skin surface and used to detect both the dynamic geometry of underlying structures (two-dimensional echo imaging) and the flow velocity within vascular structures (Doppler flowmetry). *(Center left)* an echo probe used for cardiac imaging from the surface of the body. *(Center right)* a doppler probe used for vascular flow velocity measurements from the surface of the body. *(Right)* a Doppler probe used for vascular flow velocity measurements. The miniature piezoelectric crystal is mounted within a suction cup and applied directly to the surface of the exposed vascular structure.

Applications

Echo Imaging (Ultrasound).—The rapid electrical excitation of a piezoelectric crystal produces high-frequency longitudinal shock waves (ultrasound) in the surrounding medium. These can be focused and aimed at structures in the body. The sound waves will traverse the structures in their path and are transmitted, reflected, and absorbed by those structures. If periods of excitation are alternated with periods of nonexcitation, the portion of the sound waves that is reflected back to the originating crystal will cause mechanical deformation and the production of charge in the piezo crystal. The amount of charge produced is proportional to the strength of the returning signal. More importantly, the time between the production of the original ultrasound, and the return of the reflected ultrasound is directly proportional to the distance that the sound wave traveled. That is, because sound in tissue has a known speed, the depth of structures from the ultrasound transducer can be determined by measurement of the duration between production and reception of the ultrasound.

The addition of multiarray or moving transducers, coupled with sophisticated processing and display of the reflected ultrasound signal, has allowed the acquisition of noninvasive images of moderate detail of many organs and tissues.

Dynamic Cardiovascular Dimensions.—A variation of the concept of the pulse transit time as a measurement of distance is used in the dynamic measurement of the distance between two structures. Unlike the echo principle, which uses a single crystal to both send and receive the reflected ultrasound, the pulse transit time uses two crystals placed perpendicularly to each other along a single axis. One crystal sends the ultrasound, while the other receives the transmitted ultrasound. The transit time is proportional to the distance traveled, based on the known velocity of ultrasound in tissue. The ultrasound signal is acquired at a high repetition rate which permits dynamic acquisition of dimension between the two crystals. This technique is widely used in experimental research for determination of dynamic dimensions of the heart and blood vessels.

Blood Velocity (Doppler).—The most recent biologic application of ultrasound has been the measurement of blood velocity and estimated blood flow. A reflected wave will undergo a shift from its original frequency based on the speed and direction of the object that causes the reflected wave (Doppler shift). An object heading toward the wave source will cause an increase in frequency of the reflected wave in proportion to the velocity of the source of reflection and vice versa. The source of the wave can be electromagnetic energy or sound, including ultrasound. For the Doppler measurement of speed, the piezoelectric crystal is used both as a source of ultrasound and as a receiver of reflected and frequency shifted ultrasound. The moving object that causes the Doppler shift between transmitted and reflected frequency is the red blood cell of the circulation.

This concept was originally applied to the qualitative measurement of venous flow patterns, and to the verification of the presence of blood flow in peripheral arteries. More recently, signal conditioning and display instrumentation have been used to provide a quantitative measurement of blood velocity and direction in the heart and major arteries. This information has been used to detect the presence of and degree of intracardiac shunts, determine the presence and severity of stenotic and regurgitant cardiac valve lesions, and measure the severity of stenoses in large arteries. When the flow pattern, shape, and area of a blood vessel can be determined by other methods or inference, an estimate of blood flow can be made.

Specifications
Errors.—Piezoelectric crystals have two limitations that have important implications as biologic transducers: poor low-frequency re-

sponse, and variation of the piezoelectric constant (ratio of electrical energy to mechanical force). The bandwidth of a piezoelectric crystal can be modified by selection of crystal material and by construction techniques to have a useful range from a few hertz to a few dozen megahertz. Therefore, DC and low-frequency events cannot be measured. Also, the amplitude of electrical output in response to mechanical deformation (and vice versa) of a crystal is somewhat variable and subject to environmental conditions. Therefore, measurement of amplitude response is unreliable. The history of biomedical instrumentation is littered with numerous attempts to quantitate the *amplitude* of signals obtained from piezoelectric transducers. At best, one may obtain qualitative information from instruments that were intended to measure signal amplitude, such as intensity of heart sounds and motion of apex and peripheral pulses.

The current heyday of crystal devices has been marked by recognition of their one exact quantitative feature: frequency response. Piezoelectric transducers can oscillate at exact frequencies, and electronic circuitry is available to cause crystals to oscillate with accuracy and precision and to measure this frequency of oscillation with accuracy and precision. Relieved of a quantitative amplitude response, for which they were not capable, crystals have proven themselves invaluable in ultrasound imaging and Doppler. These techniques use very high frequencies that avoid the limitations of low frequency and quantitative amplitude response.

Thermistors and Thermocouples

These devices are used for the measurement of temperature and its inferred concept of heat content. Temperature and its changes represent an important biologic characteristic. It is also of great value and interest to stimulate small and temporary changes of temperature to measure other biologic properties such as blood flow. Thermistors are active devices, whereas thermocouples are passive devices.

Thermistor
Theory.—The thermistor is based on the concept that most semiconductors change their resistance in response to temperature—as temperature goes up, resistance goes down.* This wreaks havoc with most electronic instruments and is one of the limitations on the range

---

*The opposite is true for most conductors—resistance increases as temperature increases.

of temperature operation and the stability of such instruments. However, this principle can also be harnessed for the measurement of temperature. When employed as the variable resistor as part of a bridge circuit, the resistance change of the thermistor will cause a change in the voltage output of the bridge. The voltage output of the bridge can then be calibrated in response to temperature changes.

Construction and Application.—Thermistors can be manufactured and applied in a variety of shapes and forms (Fig 5–4). Disc-like configurations are suitable for surface application, whereas tiny bead-like configurations can be mounted on the edge of a catheter. The mass of the thermistor and its surrounding and covering materials have a great effect on the time responsiveness (frequency response) of the thermistor. These properties should be determined at the time of fabrication, or can be tested before use (see chapter 9).

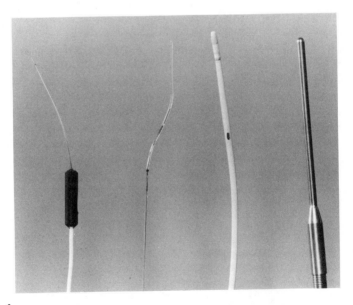

FIG 5–4.
Thermistors. A few examples of the different configurations and applications of thermistors. *(Left)* bare-tipped thermistor used for measurement of phasic respiratory temperature; the miniature size and uncovered construction allow a high frequency response needed for this particular application. *(Center)* two examples of intravascular catheter-tipped thermistors; one catheter *(center left)* contains only a thermistor; the other *(center right)* is a balloon flotation catheter containing the thermistor and ports for measurement of intravascular pressure. *(Right)* rugged thermistor used for measurement of bath temperature; the probe is placed in a fluid bath for measurement of temperature of the bath.

The rate of change of resistance of a thermistor decreases as temperature increases (Fig 5–5). Therefore, the resolution of the thermistor is better at lower than at higher temperatures. Good resolution is obtained within the biologic temperature range. The resistance change of a thermistor in response to temperature is not linear over a large temperature range, but almost linear over a narrow temperature range (e.g., a few degrees Celsius). This narrow range of temperatures is appropriate to many biologic conditions, and most thermistor applications are confined to measurement over a limited range. If used over a wider range of temperatures, a scheme for correcting this nonlinearity should be employed. In order to extend the linear range of the thermistor, electronic compensation, in the form of an analog signal processor (chapter 6), can be built into the bridge circuit, because the nonlinearities of the thermistor are known. Another way to provide correction for a nonlinear device, as long as the calibration curve is known or can be obtained, is to use a digitizing and microprocessor circuit and to compare the observed signal level to a value stored in a look-up table in computer memory (chapter 8).

Another problem of the thermistor is that a current has to be applied to the thermistor as part of the bridge circuit. Therefore, heat is generated in the thermistor while temperature is measured. It is required that either the generated heat is small or the dissipation is large in order to avoid an error in the measurement of temperature and to avoid thermal injury to the organ under observation. This limitation can be turned to an advantage. Thermistor temperature depends on the balance between heat loss and heat gain. The factors which control

FIG 5–5.

Resistance vs. temperature behavior of thermistors. This relationship is shown for three different thermistors. The scale of the vertical axis is the logarithm of the thermistor resistance at a particular temperature in reference to its resistance at 25° C. There are three themes in this diagram. First, notice that the resistance decreases as temperature increases. Second, the rate of change of resistance decreases as temperature increases (note logarithmic scale); this means that the resolution of the thermistor is better at lower than at higher temperatures. Not as obvious, because of the logarithmic scale of the diagram, is the slight nonlinearity of the resistance-to-temperature behavior of the thermistor.

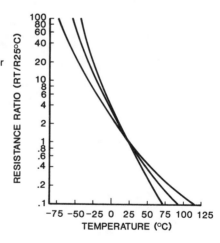

this balance are the electrical energy which is supplied to operate the thermistor, and the transfer of energy between the thermistor and the surrounding medium. If the energy supplied to the thermistor is constant, then thermistor temperature depends on heat exchange with the surrounding medium. If the thermistor is placed on a tissue surface or within a blood vessel, it is possible to calibrate such a system and measure at least relative, if not absolute, flow.

Thermocouple
Theory.—The thermocouple is a device of two dissimilar metals that produces electrical energy in proportion to the temperature at the junction of the metals. Small or galvanic currents are known to flow across the junction (the thermocouple junction) of two dissimilar metals—such as copper and constantan (a metal compound). These galvanic currents are proportional to the temperature of the junction, and for further accuracy, can be referenced to a junction of the same metals at a known temperature—usually 0° C, 100° C, or sometimes room temperature. The thermoelectric sensitivity is usually positive, that is, energy output increases as temperature increases, but is negative for some junctions. Current is converted to voltage, usually in the millivolt range, by the resistance (input impedance) of a sensing device called a galvanometer (see chapter 7).

Construction and Application.—Thermocouple junctions can be made extremely small and are known to have precise properties during manufacture and application. The usefulness of a single type of thermocouple junction is limited to about a range of 100° C; therefore, a wide variety of thermocouple junctions can be produced to cover a wide range of temperature requirements both inside and outside the biologic range. As with the thermistor, the response time of the thermocouple is governed by its mass and the type and mass of material that surrounds and supports the thermocouple. Galvanometers to assess millivolt outputs accurately were cumbersome in the past, but have now become greatly miniaturized.

Photoelectric and Scintillation Detectors

These devices are used to convert electromagnetic and radiation energy into an electrical energy output. Photoelectric detectors are commonly included in calorimeters and spectrophotometers to detect color and light absorbance of liquids and fluids and in scintillation detectors to detect light emission, while scintillation detectors are used in scintillation counters and cameras to detect the wave and particle decay of radionuclides.

Theory

The ionization effect is based on the principle that certain thin films (usually metallic) and certain crystals (notably sodium iodide) respond when exposed to electromagnetic radiation. The form of the electromagnetic radiation may be either wave or particle. If it is wave, the radiation may be light energy in the visible or invisible range (infrared or ultraviolet), or it may be radiation energy such as x-rays and gamma rays. If it is particle, the radiation may be alpha or beta particles.

Photoelectric detectors, which respond to light (visible, infrared, or ultraviolet), are categorized into three types. A detector that changes its resistance called a *photoresistor;* one that changes its voltage is called a *photovoltaic cell;* and one that produces a current is called a *photoemissive tube.* Depending on type, the output of such a detector is directed to a Wheatstone bridge, amplifier, or other signal conditioner. The characteristics vary considerably among the types (Table 5–1).

A scintillation detector produces a pulse of light in response to a source of radiation. A photoelectric detector is used as a second detector to transduce the light pulse of the scintillation cell. Its output is handled appropriate to its type.

Photoelectric Detectors

Application.—Concentrations of many molecules in solution show an inverse logarithmic relationship with transmission of light, especially light at a particular wavelength. To enhance selectivity, a specific

TABLE 5–1.

Properties of Photoelectric Detectors*

TYPE	WAVELENGTH SENSITIVITY	ACTIVE	RESPONSE TIME	LINEARITY OF RESPONSE TO LIGHT	DURABILITY
Photoemissive	Visible and blue	Yes	Short	Good	Fragile
Photovoltaic					
Photocell	Visible and	No	Longer	Nonlinear	Rugged
Photojunction	infrared	No	Short	Nonlinear	Rugged
Photoconductive					
Photoresistor	Red and	Yes	Longest	Almost	Temperature
Biased photocell	infrared	Yes	Short	Linear	sensitive
Phototransistor		Yes	Longer	Linear	but rugged

*Modified from Geddes LA, Baker LE: *Principles of Applied Biomedical Instrumentation,* ed 2. New York, John Wiley & Sons, 1975, pp 95–125.

wavelength of light is used, or a broader band of wavelengths is optically or electronically filtered to obtain a specific wavelength. A photoresistor or photovoltaic cell detects the energy of the light transmitted through the solution that contains the molecule, and changes its electrical characteristics.

For example, the oxyhemoglobin molecule demonstrates such a relationship between concentration and light transmission at 640 nm, and spectrophotometers (also called oximeters) can be constructed to measure the concentration of the oxyhemoglobin species. Light is transmitted through whole blood, or blood solutions after lysing the red cells. Since usually it is of interest to know the fractional concentration of oxyhemoglobin, it is necessary to know the concentration of oxyhemoglobin in comparison to other hemoglobin species. This is accomplished by measuring transmitted light through the hemoglobin solution at each of four wavelengths, including wavelengths specific for oxyhemoglobin, carboxyhemoglobin, methemoglobin, and total hemoglobin. In oximeters that measure only oxyhemoglobin and total hemoglobin, only two wavelengths of light are measured. The in vitro oximeter has been applied to the in vivo setting by transmission of specific wavelengths down wave guides (fiberoptics) and into vascular structures for measurement of oxygen saturation in the circulation.

Sometimes the signal of interest can be measured by creating a transducible property based on light transmission. Consider the measurement of blood volume or blood flow. Suppose one injects into the blood a substance that has unique optical transmission characteristics compared to the molecules found in blood—a dye. Colorimetric measurement of the volume (we assume it is the blood volume) in which that dye was mixed can be made by knowledge of the initial concentration (if any) of that substance in the blood volume, of the mass of the indicator molecule entered in the volume and of the final concentration of that substance in the volume. It is also possible to measure a blood volume flow rate (blood flow) by observing the time-concentration curve of the dye downstream from its site of entrance into the blood volume. These are the principles that underlie some of the methods of measurement of blood volume and cardiac output in animals and humans. This cardiac output method has almost entirely been replaced by the thermodilution method mentioned above. Note that the concepts of the two different methods for measurement of cardiac output are the same, but the transducible property (heat content vs. molecule concentration) and the signal detector (thermoelectric vs. photoelectric) are different.

Even if the compound under study does not have selective light transmission characteristics, measurement by spectrophotometry is sometimes possible. A compound with selective light wavelength absorption or emission characteristics can be introduced into the assay. This compound must bear a known relationship, that is stoichiometric, with the compound of interest undergoing chemical reaction. For example, lactate, a compound of interest in blood and tissues, has no usable wavelength absorption properties. However, its stoichiometric relationship with NAD and subsequent conversion of NAD to NADH—a compound with known wavelength absorption—allows the lactate concentration to be measured.

Errors.—There are two principle performance characteristics of a photodetector that determine the level of error. The sensitivity of a photovoltaic cell is its ability to produce an energy output in response to the energy input of the light source. A sensitivity of less than 1 would mean that output was less than input. This would produce a nonrandom error such as a bias or proportional error. The amplitude linearity of a detector is its ability to produce an energy output in proportion to energy input. A nonlinearity would mean that the gain of the system was not constant over a range of operation. This would produce a nonrandom error. In colorimetric instruments, these problems can be quite severe, but are improved in spectrophotometric instruments.

When photodetectors are used for counting or imaging, there are two additional performance characteristics that should be considered. The spatial resolution of the detector is its ability to discriminate the distance between points of light. This will determine the quality of the detail of a static image. The temporal resolution of the detector is its ability to achieve a maximal count rate. A finite time is required for the phosphor of the photodetector to recover after light strikes it. This will determine the bandwidth of the acquired data. For example, the photodetectors used in TV imaging require from about 30 to 200 msec to recover after being struck by light energy. This limits imaging rate to about 30 pictures (frames) per second.

Scintillation Detectors

Application.—The number and spatial location of radioactive particles and waves can be determined by a scintillation detector. This detector produces a scintillation (flash of light) in response to a collision with a radioactive wave or particle that releases the full or partial energy of the wave or particle. In practice, a radioactive tracer is attached to a molecule, particle, or cell and the radioactive decay products of the tracer are imaged in vitro or in vivo. The scintillation detector can be used to measure the concentration, shape, position, and motion of tagged substances and structures.

For example, it is possible to determine the presence of and the concentration, mass, or volume of substances by scintillation detectors. A sample of molecules, particles, or cells is labeled (tagged) with a radioactive tracer and mixed with the entire mass or volume of interest. The counts per minute (cpm) of the entire mass or volume, or a representative fraction of the mass or volume, are measured and compared to a known reference concentration of the radioactive tracer. This is a widely used in vitro technique in biochemistry and molecular biology. Also, radioactive tracers can be applied in vivo and counts per minute measured by externally placed scintillation detectors; or it is possible to obtain a biologic sample after in vivo administration of the radioactive tracer and to measure the counts per minute in vitro. This technique is applied widely in clinical and basic research investigations.

If the emitted particles and waves of a radioactive tracer that has been administered in vivo are collimated and observed in two or three dimensions in space, then the size and shape of the object the radioactive tracer occupies can be determined. If the dimension of time observation is added to space observation, then the motion or activity of the object the radioactive tracer occupies can be determined. This imaging technique is used widely in clinical and basic research investigations.

Errors.—There are four performance characteristics of a scintillation detector that determine the level of error. The sensitivity (also known as efficiency) of a detector is its ability to produce a scintillation (count) in response to the wave or particle produced by a radionuclide disintegration. A sensitivity less than unity would mean that output was less than input. This would produce a nonrandom error such as a bias or proportional error. In addition, counting efficiency affects image bandwidth (see below). The amplitude linearity of a detector is its ability to produce an energy output in proportion to energy input. A nonlinearity would mean that the gain of the system was not constant over a range of operation. This would produce a nonrandom error. The spatial resolution of the detector is its ability to discriminate the distance between points of radionuclide disintegration. This will determine the quality of the detail of a static image.

The temporal resolution of the detector is its ability to achieve a maximal count rate. A finite time is required for the phosphor of the scintillation detector to recover after radiation strikes it. This will determine the theoretical limit of the bandwidth of the acquired data. The current temporal resolution capabilities (>100,000 samples per second) of a scintillation detector impose no bandwidth limitation on the acquisition of most biological signals. However, there are practical limitations of instrument bandwidth based on a large number of disintegrations that have to be detected from the entire imaging field in order to have resolution of the image. This, in turn, is limited by the amount of radioactivity that can be administered and the counting efficiency. As a result, the temporal resolution capability for imaging is not limited by the counting rate of the detector, but by the required duration of the sampling of the imaging field. In humans, this limits imaging rate to about 24 frames (pictures) per second. From the Nyquist theorem (see chapter 8), the signal bandwidth is limited to no more than 12 Hz.

6

The Instrumentation Chain: II. Signal Conditioners

In this chapter we follow the signal as it is acquired from the signal detector until the stage of display and recording. This step is called *signal conditioning*, and refers to a series of (usually) interrelated steps for amplifying, filtering, and processing the acquired signal. The stereo component system, to which we referred in chapter 5, includes instruments that act as signal conditioners.

Suppose we tried to listen to the music detected by our phonograph needle as it tracked the pits and grooves on the surface of the record. Try this sometime: place your ear close to the needle and, assuming that dotage hasn't overcome your hearing threshold, you may be able to hear a faint and poor quality reproduction of the sound. This is unsatisfactory because the level of the signal is so low, it does not allow us to satisfactorily resolve the information in the sound; that is why people amplify the sound. The volume control of the stereo system is an *amplifier:* it boosts the level of the signal in order to increase the resolution of the music, and to increase the power of the signal so that the speakers of the stereo system can operate. This is also what the amplifier of a biomedical instrument does: it alters the level of the biologic signal for the purposes of increasing the resolution of the signal and for increasing the energy that is supplied to other instruments including the display device and recorder.

The bass and treble controls of the stereo system are *filters;* turning them up and down increases and decreases frequencies that are at either extreme of the musical bandwidth, the very low and the very high. We alter the level of these frequencies because it sounds better, which usually means that our knowledge of music enables us to tell which musical frequencies should be modified. This is also what the filters of a biomedical instrument do: they alter the level of some frequencies of the biologic signal because our knowledge of the signal tells us that some frequencies should be modified to provide us with more information.

The noise reduction and reverberation controls on the stereo system are *signal processors:* turning them on and off processes the musical signal and gives us some different sound than we can hear in the original music. This is also what the signal processors of a biomedical instrument do: they process the biologic signal so as to extract some important information or modify the signal so as to provide us with a novel insight.

WHAT YOU NEED TO KNOW

1. The basic electronic component of a signal conditioner is an operational amplifier. There are a number of characteristics of an op amp that affect the operation of signal conditioners.

2. An amplifier is a signal conditioner that alters the level of energy (usually increases the electrical energy) of the signal so that other instruments can process or record the signal.

3. A filter is a signal conditioner that alters the frequency content of the signal so as to remove that part of the bandwidth that is considered either irrelevant to the signal or is that part of the signal that originates from other than the intended source.

4. Signal processors are special examples of signal conditioners that perform algebraic or logical functions on the signal and are used to extract some important or interesting property of the signal that is not easily observed in its native state.

The Operational Amplifier

Probably the most ubiquitous and useful active electronic component used in instrumentation is the operational amplifier, or op amp.

An op amp does what its name implies—it operates on a signal. Originally a collection of multiple components *(discrete devices)*, the op amp has been a single component itself *(integrated circuit)* since the mid-1960s. The op amp is not an instrument itself, but rather an important electronic component of an instrument. By configuring the amplifier with different additional external components, such as resistors and capacitors, and linking multiple op amps together, it is possible to construct instruments that are capable of performing the functions discussed in the remainder of this chapter: amplifiers, filters, and signal processors. If you're not "into" electronic circuits, skip the next section.

Of all the electronic components the reader is likely to see represented by a symbol, the op amp is most prominent. It is worthwhile to look at the symbolic representation of the amplifier briefly (Fig 6–1). Typically, the triangular shaped symbol of an op amp shows the base of the triangle as its input side—the side that receives the incoming signal, while the apex of the triangle is its output side—the side that sends the operated signal on to the next electronic component. The op amp is an active device; it always requires a DC power source to operate. On most op amp symbols, these will be indicated as straight vertical lines emanating from either side of the triangle. Sometimes,

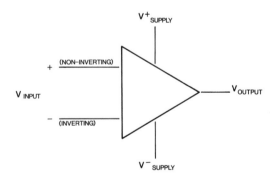

FIG 6–1.
Schematic diagram of the operational amplifier. The triangular shape represents the physical package of the amplifier. The hot or active lead of a signal referred to ground (so-called single ended) may be connected to the noninverting (+) or inverting (−) side of the amplifier. A differential signal is connected between the noninverting and the inverting inputs. If a single-ended signal enters the noninverting input side, it will be operated on and will leave the amplifier with the same polarity as it entered. If a single-ended signal enters the inverting side, it will be operated on and will leave the amplifier with its polarity inverted. Technical reasons of operation limit the use of the noninverting input side. Therefore, two op amps in series are almost always used to "correct" the signal to its original polarity. Power supply connections for a DC source (V^+ *supply* and V^- *supply*) are optionally indicated on a schematic; however, because the op amp is an active device, a power supply is always required.

these lines are missing, but they are always implied. You'll recall from chapter 1 that a part of each instrument package containing electrical and electronic components is devoted to converting AC power from the "power main" (AC line circuit) to DC in order to power the components of the instrument. The op amp represents one of the major components that strictly requires DC voltage and current, and its function depends on the consistency of this power supply.

The ideal operational amplifier would have the following characteristics: infinite gain, no offset bias, no input current, infinite input impedance, and no output impedance. We will discuss the meaning and practical limitation of these specifications as we examine the instrumentation amplifier in the following section.

The Amplifier

An amplifier receives a signal input from a signal detector or signal processor, and provides an altered signal level (usually increased) as its output. From the user's standpoint, amplifiers are usually inconspicuous because one doesn't directly connect them to a patient, and does not directly observe their output. However, amplifiers serve a vital function in the instrument chain.

Why Amplify?

The energy level of biologic signals is quite small. Although the adult human body at rest produces the power equivalent of about 75 watts, certainly enough if harnessed to energize a light bulb, the energy is diversely and diffusely consumed by many different processes in many different parts of the body. The energy production of an organ, tissue, or cell is correspondingly less. Even if we could tap into this energy source (as horror filmmakers have suggested, usually for some evil purpose) there would be less available to maintain the integrity and function of the body. Therefore, it is not surprising that the energy level of a signal that is transmitted from the biologic system to the outside world is usually small. There are exceptions to this: if we were to transduce the motion of another person's good swift kick by one of our sensorineural endings, we might well be aware of its energy content on our shin or elsewhere.

Although a signal detector alters the form of the native signal, say from ionic to galvanic electrical current (electrode) or from pressure to resistance (strain gauge transducer), it won't increase the energy content of the signal. The limitation in the transfer of a transduced biologic signal along the instrument chain is that instruments of the chain require a higher signal energy than can be provided by the native signal. This higher signal energy is required in order to (1) increase the resolution of different levels of the signal, and (2) operate other instruments in the chain that require high signal power.

An amplifier provides this increase in signal energy by taking the signal from the electrode or transducer at its input and increasing (amplifying) the energy of the signal at its output for use by other instruments. Typically, the voltage level of output of a signal detector is in the microvolt to millivolt range (a so-called low-level signal), whereas display devices and recorders operate at a level of a few volts (a so-called high-level signal). Ultimately, this increase in energy must be provided by one or more stages of amplification.

Classes of Amplifiers.—There are two broad classes of amplifiers: instrumentation and power (driver) amplifier. The principal purpose of an instrumentation amplifier is to increase the voltage of the signal so that resolution of the signal can be increased. An instrumentation amplifier receives a low level (low voltage—microvolt to millivolt range) signal from the transducer or electrode and increases the voltage (volt range) of the signal. The principal purpose of a power amplifier is to increase the power of the signal so that it will operate or drive another instrument which requires high power. A power amplifier receives a high level (volt range) signal from an instrumentation amplifier and increases the power of the signal in order to drive the operation of a recorder.

Amplifier Specifications
These specifications define the performance of the amplifier.

Sensitivity.—The sensitivity, gain, or amplification of a system is the ratio of its output to its input, expressed in the dimensions of the output and input (Fig 6–2). If we are referring to an instrumentation amplifier, both the input and output of the amplifier will be in the same electrical units, either voltage or current. Thus, sensitivity becomes a dimensionless ratio such as $\times 10$ (read this as *times 10*), $\times 250$, or $\times 1,000$. For example, if the instrumentation amplifier input was 1 mV, then the output would be 0.01, 0.25, or 1 V, respectively. On the other hand, the output of a power or driver amplifier is frequently directed to an oscilloscope or writing recorder. In that case, the output becomes a deflection of a light beam or the movement of a pen or tracing on a paper. The sensitivity of such a system is specified as 'x' cm output (deflection of beam implied) per 'y' voltage level of signal

FIG 6–2.
Sensitivity or gain of an amplifier.
Sensitivity is the ratio of output to input. In
an instrumentation amplifier, both input and
output are measured in terms of voltage
and sensitivity is a nondimensional ratio.
The output of detectors used for biologic
signals is commonly at the millivolt or
microvolt level. In order to improve signal
resolution and to operate other instruments
in the instrumentation chain, this low-level
signal is typically amplified to the level of
about a volt.

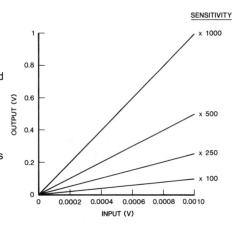

input. Sometimes, the inverse of this figure is reported as the sensitivity: 'x' voltage level input per 'y' cm output. For example, the driver amplifier on my recorder has increasing levels of sensitivity from 1,000 mv/cm to 1 mv/cm.

There is a practical limitation to the level of sensitivity of an amplifier. However, it is possible and frequently necessary to place multiple stages of amplification in series (one amplifier receives as its input the output of another amplifier) in order to achieve very high levels of gain that would not be practical in a single stage.

There may be *error* associated with sensitivity. Amplifier sensitivity may not be a constant, but may vary over a range of static and dynamic (frequency components) inputs. The amount of this variation over the input range may be expressed as the maximum deviation of the sensitivity of the amplifier from a nominal value. However, the variation of amplifier sensitivity is usually calculated as a type of RMS value over the entire range of input. This is called the *total harmonic distortion* (THD), which is expressed as a percentage of the signal output, such as 1% THD.

Range.—There is a limitation of the maximum level of signal that can be produced as output of the amplifier. This is called the amplifier output saturation voltage. Typically, the amplifier output saturation voltage might be 1, 5, or 12 V or (rarely) higher. The usual limitation to the saturation voltage of an amplifier is the actual voltage supply level at which it is operated. The maximum signal voltage output of an amplifier cannot exceed its supply voltage, that is, the voltage of the energy source that powers the operation of the amplifier. However, it is rarely necessary to increase the level of signal output of an amplifier beyond a few volts, because most instruments downstream in the instrumentation chain have a maximum signal input limitation of a few volts.

There are *errors* due to range. There is an interaction between the level of the input to the amplifier, its sensitivity or gain, and its output saturation voltage. For example, consider an amplifier that has a maximum output of 1 V. An input signal that had a level of 1 mV could be amplified with any of the gains cited in the previous paragraph, yet its output would not exceed 1 V. However, if the input signal were 20 mV, only sensitivities up to ×500 could be used before the amplifier output would be saturated, because the voltage of the input signal multiplied by the sensitivity equals the voltage output (20 mV × 500 = 1 V). The usual result of saturating the output of an amplifier is clipping of the output—the signal input may increase, but the output assumes a fixed, maximum value.

Input Offset and Suppression.—There frequently is a bias at the input of an amplifier. That is, there may be a DC level different from zero even when the signal level is zero. This offset may be introduced by the signal itself, or by an earlier instrument in the chain, or by the amplifier itself (input bias of the amplifier). If this bias occurs at the input to the amplifier, the amplifier increases (amplifies) the level of both the bias and the true level of the signal. This problem especially occurs with low-level signals and high amplifier sensitivity.

At first look, the user might be satisfied that an amplifier with a maximum output voltage specification of 1 V could handle any small input signal contaminated by a bias without becoming saturated regardless of the level of sensitivity. But that is just not so. Any offset that is present at the input of an amplifier can saturate the amplifier output at sufficiently high sensitivity (Fig 6–3). If the signal offset is not removed the maximum usable level of amplification will be reduced. This may be handled in two ways: AC coupling (which is actually high-pass filtering) which removes all DC levels including the mean of the signal and its input bias (see below), or input suppression. This latter method is used if important information about the signal is contained in its average or DC level, but bias needs to be removed. In that case, a voltage of opposite polarity to the bias is summed with the incoming signal before it reaches the amplifier to remove it or to "buck" it out.

For example, consider an amplifier that has an output saturation voltage of 1 V. The maximum sensitivity that could be applied to a

FIG 6–3.

Limitation of input offset on amplifier sensitivity. An amplifier increases the level of all input—both the true signal and offset (also called bias). Limitation of the level of output *(maximum output)* requires limitation of any source of offset. Here it is shown that when offset is any fraction of signal input, the maximum sensitivity that can be applied to the input signal is severely reduced. For example, the limit of amplification is only ×5 when input offset is 20% of maximum amplifier output. As input offset progressively falls toward zero, the theoretical limit of amplification of the desired signal input increases toward infinity. In practice, maximum sensitivity is not infinite, but is limited by the properties of the electronic components of the amplifier.

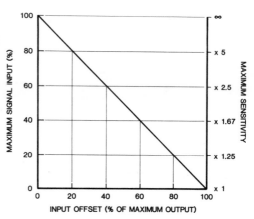

signal that had a bias of 0.1 V would be ×10 before saturating the amplifier. Now suppose the signal of interest was only 1 mV, riding on top of this bias. During amplification the level of the signal of interest would become overwhelmed by the much greater level of the amplified bias signal, and we wouldn't greatly improve our resolution of the low-level signal. We would be effectively observing an amplified signal of 10 mVs out of a total amplified output of 1 V. In order to correct this bias error, an adjustable amplifier suppression voltage of opposite sign to that of the bias is constantly applied to the input of the amplifier (in this case, −0.1 V) to cancel the input bias, without interfering with the relative changes of the signal level. If this suppression is entirely successful, it would restore our ability to use an amplifier sensitivity of up to ×1,000 to increase signal resolution.

There can be *errors* associated with input offset. If the added offset is itself too large, it will not only cancel the input bias, but also create its own input bias that may swamp the output capacity of the amplifier; this also will result in clipping.

Input Mode.—Amplifiers are specified according to the mode of the input signal as either single-ended or differential.

A single-ended signal has one hot or active pole whose voltage is referenced to ground. Signal voltages may be either positive or negative with reference to ground (unipolar input) or both (bipolar input). A single-ended amplifier may be designed to accept either unipolar or bipolar signals: a bipolar amplifier can accept either type of voltage input, whereas a unipolar amplifier cannot. They are commonly used as a latter stage in a series of amplifiers or in simple amplification situations where a high-level, low-noise signal is available. Because of its electronic construction, a single-ended amplifier cannot be used as a differential amplifier.

A differential amplifier amplifies the signal difference between the two poles of the input. Coincidentally, one of these poles might be at ground potential, but usually they are not. The output of most signal detectors (electrodes, crystal devices, and transducers) is not referenced to ground because a signal is produced as a result of a voltage differential between two electrode leads, across the crystal, or between the active arms of a strain gauge bridge. For example, when measured by an electrode pair, a cellular bioelectric potential of -90 mV represents the voltage difference between the inside referenced to the outside of the cell, and not to absolute reference level of ground. Similarly, the voltage potential of about 1 mV of the R wave of lead I of the human electrocardiogram is generated as the voltage potential between the left arm and the right arm, without reference to ground.

Differential amplifiers have two inputs: one labeled "+" and the other labeled "−", or perhaps labeled as accepting two specific leads from a signal detector, if the amplifier is dedicated to a particular measurement. Admittedly, this can be somewhat confusing. There is an apocryphal story of a well-known Chief of Cardiology who, when he was a fellow, couldn't understand how an amplifier labeled "ECG amplifier" could be used to measure a signal other than an electrocardiogram. The answer is that an ECG amplifier is a differential amplifier that, if constructed in a flexible configuration, will accept a differential input from a variety of sources. A differential amplifier can also be used as a single-ended amplifier by physically attaching the "−" lead on the input port to ground, or by supplying an input signal that is single-ended—that is, already referenced to ground.

Common Mode Rejection.—One of the significant advantages of a differential amplifier is the signal-to-noise ratio enhancement obtained by common mode rejection of noise. Signal interference (noise) may occur at the site of the generation of the biologic signal, on its way into the instrument (cable or connector) or within the instrument itself. In a differential amplifier, any noise that occurs on both of the input leads *(in common)* will be rejected in favor of the true signal—that is, the signal not in common on the two leads.

How does the differential amplifier do this? Because common noise occurs on both the noninverting ("+") and the inverting ("−") inputs of the amplifier, the differential amplifier will sum both the noise signal and the inverted noise signal. They will cancel, and therefore noise will not appear at the output of the amplifier, while the true differential signal will appear amplified at the output (Fig 6–4). One usual source of signal in common is the 60 Hz electrical interference ("power mains noise"), which is ubiquitous wherever there is power line wiring and electrical equipment.

The specification for common mode rejection is given as the quotient of a difference in signal between the two inputs to that which appears in common between the two inputs: the common mode rejection ratio (CMRR). Typically, this number will be 10,000 to 100,000 to 1 or greater (80 to 100 dB; Fig 6–5). Single-ended amplifiers do not provide common mode rejection because they have only one active pole, while the other input is connected to an electrically neutral point "ground."

Input and Output Impedance.—The power transfer characteristics of an amplifier—its relationship to the source that feeds the input signal to the amplifier, and its relationship to the device that will receive the output from the amplifier—are expressed as the input and output impedance of the amplifier. The amplifier should be a selfless instrument; it should take as little energy as possible from the input, and provide as much energy as possible at the output. In this discussion, it is necessary to separate the electrical power supply requirements of the amplifier from its signal power input and output specification; it is the latter which we are discussing. As a biologic analogy, one separates

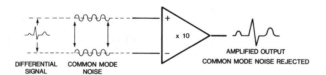

FIG 6–4.

Common mode rejection. A differential amplifier receives at its input both signal and noise. The signal is a voltage difference between the two poles of the input, while the noise appears the same ("in common") on both poles. The common mode noise, which may be many times greater than the level of the signal, is rejected while the signal is amplified.

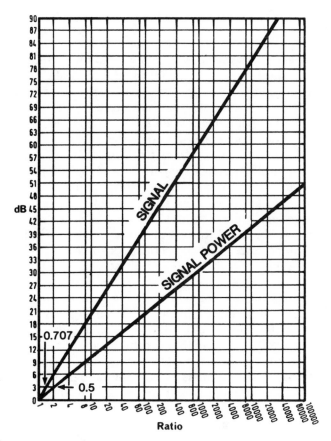

FIG 6–5.

The decibel diagram. When there is a large range of ratios, engineers frequently express this range as a logarithmic scale called the decibel, or dB. A dB for acoustical signals is calculated as ten times the $\log_{10}$ of the ratio. A dB for electronic signals is calculated as 20 times the $\log_{10}$ for voltage or current, and ten times the $\log_{10}$ for power. Among frequently mentioned decibel values in this book is 3 dB. For a voltage or current signal, this would correspond to a fraction of 0.707. For a power signal, this would correspond to a fraction of 0.5. The two numbers that compose the ratio can come from any source whose ratio is appropriate to compare. The arrangement of the two numbers into either the numerator or the denominator of the ratio depends entirely on the context of the discussion. In this book, the numerator is the output level of an instrument at a particular frequency, whereas the denominator is the output level at the flat portion of the bandwidth of the instrument. Therefore, the ratio compares the instrument output at a specified frequency compared to a reference frequency.

cardiac metabolism (the power supply requirements of the heart) from cardiac input and output (the mechanical performance specifications of the heart).

There are errors associated with a low-input impedance, and therefore input impedance should be kept as high as possible (typically 1 to 10 megohms or more). There are three concrete reasons for this. First, it is important not to load down the source of the input signal. Biologic signal sources or signal detectors can be considered as limited current sources. This signal input current is converted to a voltage at the input of the amplifier by the resistance of the leads that carry the signal in series with the input resistance (impedance) of the amplifier ($E = I \times R$). A low input resistance may cause an input current load in excess of signal capacity, and the result is that signal voltage will fall—the level will be reduced. For a number of reasons, it is preferred not to add resistance to the input leads, but rather to have an amplifier with a high input impedance. Second, because of these loading effects, input impedance may alter the level and phase of the frequency components of a signal and this may cause distortion of the signal, similar to the effects of nonlinearities of sensitivity mentioned above. A high input impedance will minimize distortion. Third, input impedance will have effects on the apparent CMRR. A high input impedance will maintain the CMRR of an amplifier near to its specification.

Output impedance determines the power output capabilities of the amplifier. Although all amplifiers should have a high input impedance, it is only necessary for amplifiers that connect directly to other instruments that have a large energy requirement (such as a pen writing recorder) to have a low output impedance. Because integrated circuits tolerate only low voltage, high power output is achieved through high current output, rather than high voltage output ($P = I \times V$).

Frequency Response or Bandwidth.—This amplifier specification defines that portion of the signal frequency spectrum that will be amplified by the instrument. The principles of the bandwidth are the same for an amplifier as they are for a signal detector: the object is to pass the level and phase of all the frequency content of the signal without alteration. The catch is that technology has not been able to deliver the amplifier of infinite bandwidth, and that biologic signals and instrument errors sometimes require limitation of bandwidth. There are considerations at both ends of the bandwidth—the high- and low-frequency components.

To some extent, the discussion of amplification of high-frequency components of the bandwidth has historical value. It required a number of generations of electronic components to achieve amplifiers that had an adequate high-frequency response. This is no longer a problem with the *design* of amplifiers used in biology, where high-frequency response need not exceed 10,000 Hz, and is usually much lower; but limited high-frequency response is still very problematic with the mechanical devices of which transducers and recorders are constructed. However, there are problems in the *use* of a wide bandwidth amplifier with respect to sources of error. Forms of random error (noise) from the amplifier itself are present at all frequencies. The wider the bandwidth, the greater the noise. Because the bandwidth-to-total noise relationship is not linear, it's especially beneficial to limit the very-high-frequency response. In addition, noise from extraneous sources with a high-frequency content (biologic or physical), may contaminate the signal of interest. Therefore, it pays to limit the high-frequency portion of the bandwidth to that of the signal of interest so as to avoid the unnecessary introduction of noise.

Similarly, the physical capability of design and construction of amplifiers with a very-low-frequency response has only recently been surmounted with the development of discrete devices; however, application of very-low-frequency response amplifiers still poses problems with some signals, as we will discuss next.

Coupling.—Amplifiers are either AC or DC coupled. Despite the common terminology with electrical power, this has nothing to do with power supply, but rather input signal. AC-coupled amplifiers block DC, but amplify any non-steady portion of the input signal—they behave like a high pass filter (see below).

As discussed previously (chapter 2) the frequency spectrum provides the investigator with information about the presence and quantitative importance of the high-frequency components of the signal. Practically speaking, this translates into instrument bandwidth requirements. But the Fourier spectrum does not always provide us with practical information about the very-low-frequency components. The frequency spectrum includes a mean or DC (zero frequency, by analogy with electrical power terminology) component term of each signal frequency spectrum, which would indicate that the bandwidth for the proper recording of a signal should go down as low as DC. However, for many signals the information of interest is found in the variations of the signal and not the average or DC value. For example, the variations and not the DC bioelectrical activity of whole organs and tissues (like the heart, brain, and muscle) are commonly of interest to the observer. Furthermore, practical considerations in the application and design of instruments dictate that it is not always beneficial or possible for instruments to have a bandwidth that goes as low as DC.

Until recently, it was not possible to construct high-gain DC amplifiers—that is, amplifiers whose bandwidth ranged down to 0 Hz. Of greater importance is the presence of some forms of instrument error such as electrode noise and amplifier drift, which we discussed in chapter 3. One would quickly run out of offset capability and patience constantly adjusting the offset of many signals that have these errors. AC-coupled amplifiers will block or remove part or all of these low-frequency signals if their frequency content is below that of the specification of the amplifier.

The limitation of AC-coupled amplifiers is that one can only measure a change in the level of a signal, and not its absolute or DC level. In contrast, DC-coupled amplifiers are intended to amplify absolute voltage levels; that is, they report both steady-state and non–steady-state aspects of a signal. DC amplifiers are applicable where the rate and magnitude of drift is very small compared to the level and the duration of observation of the biologic signal. Exactly what is tolerable depends on the intent and duration of the experiment.

The Amplifier as a Physical Package.—The above information was meant to provide the reader with the concepts and the specifications of amplifier operation. The amplifier as an instrument package offers the opportunity to see how theory is put into practice. There is little application in a biologic laboratory for a fixed-gain, wide bandwidth amplifier. In my laboratory we do find occasional use for such small instrument packages to perform a single and defined task, and these can be readily constructed as needed. Rather, commercial instrumentation amplifiers usually include multiple functions housed in a single package.

One example of an amplifier is the strain gauge amplifier. This instrumentation amplifier usually has a multiconnector plug that both carries power to a strain gauge (pressure transducer) in order to energize the transducer bridge and receives signal from the strain gauge. Additionally, the transducer signal may be amplified at either a fixed or variable sensitivity. Some zero suppression adjustment will also be present. Another example of a multifunction amplifier is an all-purpose instrumentation amplifier. The amplifier is suitable for low-level signal input in the differential mode, or for high-level signal input in the single-ended mode. It has provision for changing the input mode from DC to AC coupled, and for amplifying at various levels of sensitivity. There may be zero suppression capability for the DC-coupled mode. In the AC-coupled mode it may be used as an ECG amplifier with provision to switch between different pairs of leads.

Another example of an amplifier is the oscilloscope or recorder amplifier. This power amplifier usually plugs directly into or is an integral part of the oscilloscope or recorder. Its function is to increase the power of a signal in order to drive another component that is power intensive, such as the galvanometer of the recorder. It will receive the signal from an instrumentation amplifier, and pass on the signal to the recorder with increased power. The amplifier will have adjustable levels of sensitivity, indicated as 'y' units of output signal deflection per 'x' units of input signal (either voltage or a dimension of a specific signal, such as mm Hg). Some zero suppression adjustment will also be present.

Some amplifiers are dedicated to a single purpose, and one finds both a label on the amplifier and a connecting plug that has but a single function, such as an ECG amplifier. But keep in mind that the electronic circuitry of an ECG amplifier is essentially that of a differential input and AC-coupled amplifier. It is the manufacturer who has chosen to limit the flexibility of application. Some amplifiers have signal processing and filtering capabilities that can be adjusted by the user. We will now turn our attention to these functions.

Filters

Signal filtering is the elimination of part of the frequency content of the signal. One of the mandatory features of instrumentation (including transducers, amplifiers, and recorders) is the ability not to alter the bandwidth of the signal. Filters seemingly have an inverse role—the elimination of part of the bandwidth.

Why Filter?

If the goal of instrumentation is the unaltered transfer of the information contained in the signal along the instrumentation chain, then why "blow it" with a filter? The answer is that sometimes frequency components are contained in signals that have no important information content. Filtering limits part of the bandwidth of the acquired signal, but when applied correctly it does not limit the bandwidth containing the actual signal of interest.

Transducers and signal detectors may not have perfect selectivity; that is, they may admit more than the desired signal. The source of these signals may be biologic or nonbiologic in origin. As an example, 50 to 60 Hz line power noise is broadly present in the environment and is further generated by capacitive coupling within the signal cable and the instrument case of most line-powered equipment. This undesirable information, or "noise," may be reduced by signal filtering. If the signal is differential, it is actually far more preferable to use the common mode rejection properties of a differential amplifier to reduce common mode noise.

The Ideal Filter

A filter has a corner frequency that distinguishes what part of the frequency content is to be removed, and what part is to remain. Ideally, there would be a sharp threshold: on one side the frequencies would "pass" while on the other side the frequencies would be rejected. What would happen if a signal encountered such a device? All the frequencies allowed in the pass band of the filter would go merrily zipping through, while the others would be rejected. The output signal would be reconstructed from the pass band and would appear as a signal that had frequencies removed.

Filters are broadly classified into three groups (Fig 6–6). If the filter permits the passage of all frequencies above a certain frequency level, it is called a *high-pass* filter. If the filter permits the passage of all frequencies below a certain frequency level, it is called a *low-pass* filter. If the filter permits the passage of a range of frequencies between some upper and lower frequency level, it is called a *bandpass* filter. It is not possible to construct an analog filter that has this ideal characteristic of

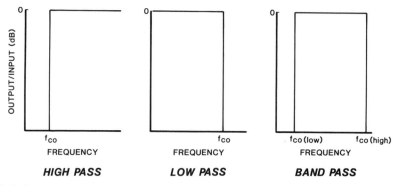

FIG 6–6.
Ideal filters. Ideally, a filter would make a very sharp discrimination between frequencies that would pass and those that would be rejected. A high-pass filter passes all "high" frequencies; that is, those frequencies *above* its corner (f_{co}). A low-pass filter passes all "low" frequencies *below* its f_{co}. A bandpass filter acts as a high pass and low pass in series, and passes a band of frequencies between the high and low f_{co}'s.

absolute threshold because of the behavior of the devices that are used to construct the filter. Digital filters—that is, filters that are a set of instructions that are executed on a digital computer and that operate on digital data—can much more closely approximate this ideal. They are discussed in chapter 8.

How an Analog Filter Works

For those with a healthy curiosity, here's how a filter works. You don't really need this to understand how to use a filter (you can skip right to the next section), but it could make you the center of attention at your next cocktail party.

You'll recall from chapter 1 that capacitors and inductors can exhibit dissipative properties much like resistors. The difference is that this resistance-like property (called *reactance*) depends on the frequency of the signal that is passed through the storage device. A capacitor entirely blocks DC or 0 frequency signals, but shows progressively less reactance at higher frequencies. Its exact level of behavior depends on its capacitance: the greater the capacitance the lower the reactance at any given frequency. The opposite is true of inductors. An inductor entirely passes DC but shows increasingly greater reactance at higher frequencies. Its exact level of behavior depends on its inductance: the greater the inductance the higher the reactance at any given frequency. Perhaps this can be remembered as, "an inductor is reluctant to pass high frequencies—a capacitor has the capacity to do so."

This variable reactance property is at the heart of how an analog filter works. If one connects one of these storage elements to a resistor, and connects one end of this combination to a signal source and the other end to ground, an interesting series of yin-yang events occurs at the point or where the two elements are joined (Fig 6–7). If the capacitor end of a combination is joined to a signal source and the resistor end to ground, the signal level at the node connecting capacitor to resistor will be zero at a DC frequency (the capacitor has infinite resistance at 0 frequency). If frequencies above zero are encountered, the voltage at the node will progressively increase to a maximum as the reactance of the capacitor falls with increasing frequency of the signal. An inductor and resistor arranged opposite to the described arrangement would behave similarly. In essence, we have created a high-pass filter: a filter that blocks DC and blocks low-frequency components to some extent.

If a capacitor and resistor are rearranged so that the resistor is attached to the signal source and the capacitor is attached to ground, the opposite effect is encountered (Fig 6–7). At DC and low frequencies,

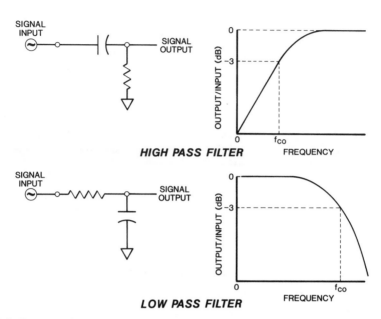

FIG 6–7.
Simple practical filters. Analog filters are based on the frequency-dependent properties of reactances (inductors and capacitors). A simple high-pass filter may be constructed from a series capacitor and a parallel resistor. The series capacitor blocks frequencies less completely as frequency increases. A simple low-pass filter may be constructed from a series resistor and a parallel capacitor. The parallel capacitor blocks frequencies more completely as frequency increases. Note that in contrast to the ideal filter, the real filter somewhat gradually discriminates between which frequencies are passed and which are rejected. The term "cutoff" (f_{co}) is used to describe that frequency which more or less discriminates between what is passed and what is rejected. At the cutoff frequency, signal level has already been reduced 3 dB (to 70.7%) of its input level.

the capacitor acts as an infinite resistor, none of the voltage can pass across it to ground, and the full signal appears at the node connecting the elements. However, at higher frequencies, the reactance of the capacitor falls, and voltage is shunted to ground. Therefore, progressively less of the signal appears at the node between the two elements. An inductor and a resistor arranged opposite to that described here would behave in the same manner. In essence, we have created a low-pass filter: a filter that blocks high-frequency components and allows some low-frequency components to pass.

The Real Filter

Real filters depart from ideal filters in two important ways. Because there is no absolute threshold of filter function, a new term called the *cutoff frequency* is introduced to describe the point of effective action. Also, because there is no cliff of activity, but at best a steep hill, the term *roll-off* is used to describe activity.

Cutoff Frequency.—For analog filters, there is a gentle reduction of the level of the signal as it moves from the flat portion of the filter bandwidth into what ideally would be the corner frequency. Therefore, rather than describing a filter by this term, it is more customary to describe a cutoff frequency whose definition is the point at which signal level is reduced 3 dB, which means that the remaining signal has been reduced to a level of 70.7% of the original. It is customary to express the pass band of a transducer, amplifier, filter, or signal processor (but not a recorder) as those frequencies between the upper and lower cutoff frequencies.

For example, a high-pass filter that has a cutoff frequency of 0.05 Hz (commonly used for human ECG studies) has already reduced the level of an input signal containing that frequency to 70.7% of its original level. Consistent with the function of this high-pass filter, higher frequency components are reduced less, and lower frequency components are reduced more. As another example, a low-pass filter that has a cutoff frequency of 100 Hz (also commonly encountered in human physiologic studies) has already reduced the level of an input signal containing that frequency to 70.7% of its original level. Consistent with the function of this low-pass filter, higher frequency components are reduced more, while lower frequency components are reduced less.

At what frequency does the filtering stop; that is, where on the pass band do you leave the signal alone compared to what happens at the cutoff frequency? The signal level increases very slowly between the cutoff and the unaltered part of the pass band. In general, the unaltered portion of the band is at a frequency that is a factor of 20 away from the cutoff. For the high-pass filter cited above, frequencies of 1 Hz and higher are passed without any reduction of signal level. Between 1 Hz and the cutoff of 0.05 Hz there is progressive reduction of the level down 3 dB. For the low-pass filter cited above, frequencies of 5 Hz and lower are passed without any reduction of level. Between 5 Hz and the cutoff at 100 Hz there is progressive reduction of the level down 3 dB. The cutoff frequency is an important milestone, because reduction of signal level gets a lot stiffer on the other side of the cutoff due to roll-off.

Roll-off.—What happens to frequencies on the other side of the cutoff away from the pass band is a progressive reduction of signal level. The steepness or slope of this reduction depends on the components of the filter. For a simple resistor-capacitor (or inductor) electrical device described previously, the roll-off is 3 dB for every time the frequency changes by a factor of 2 (an octave). That is, beyond the cutoff frequency the signal level is reduced to 70.7% of its existing level for every octave change in frequency. For the high-pass filter cited above, as frequency decreases from 0.05 Hz to 0.025 Hz (an octave), signal level decreases an additional 3 dB. This would bring the total signal reduction at 0.025 Hz to 50% (0.707 × 0.707). This continues as frequency is progressively halved, or if you're coming up the slope, as frequency is doubled. For the low-pass filter cited above, as frequency increases from 100 Hz to 200 Hz, signal level decreases down to 50% of that observed for frequencies on the flat portion of the pass band.

This is not an efficient reduction, especially compared to our expectations based on the ideal filter. One could connect multiple RC networks together for greater filter effect, but this will load down the level of the signal—even the level of the signal in the passband will be reduced. This is where the op amp comes in. By connecting the RC filter network to one or more op amps, one creates an active filter that, while it does not alter the general concepts of cutoff and roll-off, greatly increases the steepness of the roll-off without decreasing the signal level of the pass band. It is possible and frequently desirable to achieve roll-offs of 6, 12, or 24 dB per octave. Therefore, one more sharply defines the differences between frequencies included and excluded in the bandwidth of the filter. However, this improvement is taken advisedly because of the large level of signal that still appears with frequencies around the cutoff, and the somewhat reduced signal level that appears between the cutoff and the flat portion of the pass band.

The Filter as a Physical Package

Because filters are not conspicuously labeled as such on many instrument packages, they are more likely than not to cause confusion and inappropriate use when encountered. The user will most likely find filters incorporated as part of instrumentation amplifiers. Just consider the package as two separate instruments: the amplifier and the filter. If the amplifier has an AC-coupled mode along with a filter, then filter settings suitable for a high-pass filter must be used in this mode. In the DC-coupled mode, it is only possible to use a low-pass filter, because the DC mode is intended to pass the 0 and ultralow frequency components of the signal.

In either case, the user needs to remember that the filter settings supplied are those of the cutoff: signal level is already reduced at the cutoff frequency. If this frequency contains important signal information, then a setting should be chosen that is away from this frequency. Sometimes one has to compromise between removing a frequency component that has a small magnitude and allowing frequencies that represent noise to enter the instrument chain. This is especially true of low-pass filters and biologic signals. The Fourier spectrum of many of these signals shows high frequencies of very low amplitude which, although they are present, contribute little to the information content of the signal. It is possible that at frequencies just above this, there are noise components. One is frequently faced with tough choices as to whether to include these small component frequencies and risk the inclusion of noise, or whether to filter the noise and eliminate some of the frequency content of the signal. There is no easy answer to this.

One application of a filter is to limit the high-frequency error signals that other instruments introduce into the instrumentation chain. For example, transducers may introduce error signals due to resonance (chapter 3), or amplifiers may introduce Johnson or thermal noise (chapter 9). In general it is not possible to prevent these errors of the transducer or amplifier—you generally have to take whatever output it gives you. However, it is possible to consider the use of a filter to remove these signals, although there are limitations to this type of filtering. Unless the frequency of the noise is substantially higher than the frequencies of the biologic signal, one risks filtering the bandwidth of the signal along with the noise.

Filter specifications for roll-off are rarely included on the settings of the filter. Some filters will indicate that they can be set in the RC mode (i.e., 3 dB/octave) or at some higher roll-off. If this is not indicated, then chances are only a single roll-off slope exists for that instrument, but one is not sure what that is without consulting the device specifications page in the instrument manual.

Signal Processors

Signal processors are used in parallel to the instrument chain to perform some mathematical function on the signal. These devices are labor saving in that their function reduces the amount of effort required for post processing of the signal and for analysis. Because they make their information available during data acquisition, they can also assist in decision making during data collection. Their output is usually directed to some display or recording device. The most frequent use of a signal processor is to average, integrate, or differentiate the signal (Fig 6–8).

A wide variety of other logical and mathematical operations is possible with analog signal processors. Signal processing can also be elegantly performed by a digital computer (see chapter 8).

Signal Mean

The mean or average of the signal level may have biologic significance, such as the mean arterial pressure. Signal mean can be obtained in two ways. As shown in the Fourier transform, the signal mean is really the zero harmonic or DC level of the signal. This suggests that the signal mean can be obtained from an ultra-low-pass filter whose cutoff frequency is set near the frequency that corresponds to the first harmonic (the inverse of the period of the signal). The signal output will be directly available as a continuous output, but it must be appreciated that a filter will not deliver a smooth DC level as the mean; there will be some fluctuation. Also there is a time delay between the actual signal and the observed mean of the signal due to a phase shift of the signal. Another method for obtaining the signal mean involves measuring the integral of the signal (see below).

Signal Integral

The area under the curve of a signal, that is, the area that can be found between the level of the signal and some reference level (usually

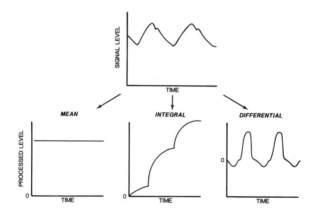

FIG 6–8.
Examples of common signal processors. A conceptual signal is shown in the top panel. The lower panels show the conditioned result of processing the mean *(left)*, the integral *(center)*, and the differential *(right)*.

ground in a single-ended signal or baseline in a differential signal) can be integrated. Electronically this is accomplished by having an amplifier feed the signal output to a storage device such as a capacitor. The capacitor continuously stores all levels of the signal and therefore integrates the area under the signal. Signal integration finds application during many biochemical assays where the value is dependent on the area under an activity curve. In physiologic signals, the integral is used in the measurement of cardiac output by the indicator dilution method. Some applications require the signal mean to be measured over a period of time; although the filter technique described above is best used for observing the mean signal in a continuous manner, more discrete measurement of the mean signal over a time epoch can be obtained by integrating the signal over the epoch, and dividing that integral by the exact duration of the epoch. This technique is commonly used in determination of minute ventilation in respiratory physiology.

Signal Differential

Signal differentiation is the mathematical function of measuring the rate of change of a signal over time. Electronically, differentiation is the inverse of signal integration. The differentiator responds only to a change of signal level, and not to the absolute level of the signal. In terms of frequency, the differentiator gives a rising output with increasing frequency. In some respects, the differentiator behaves like the slope of a high-pass filter where the cutoff frequency is set quite low so as to allow any frequency above DC to pass. Differentiation of the signal with respect to time is used in studies of electrical signals to characterize the rate of electrical processes including rates of membrane depolarization and estimates of conduction velocity. In this application, differentiation is called slew rate (dV/dt). In hemodynamics, differentiation with respect to time of left ventricular pressure rise is a reflection of shortening properties of the ventricle (dp/dt).

There are two limitations related to frequency response in the application of differentiation. First, although an ideal differentiator has no limitation of frequency response, a real differentiator does. A differentiator should increase its output level in proportion to frequency, but a real differentiator has a cutoff frequency at which point output does not increase any further despite an increase in frequency of the signal. Therefore, the investigator has to know the bandwidth of the differentiator with respect to signal bandwidth. This brings us to the second limitation: the frequency content of a differentiated signal includes higher frequencies than the signal itself. Information on differentiated signal bandwidth is rarely available; and, it is inappropriate to use the bandwidth of the signal itself to estimate the bandwidth of the differentiated signal. However, it is possible to obtain this information from further analysis of the Fourier spectrum of the signal.

Other Mathematical Operations

In addition to the above, other useful operations may be performed by a signal processor. The four basic mathematical functions (multiplication, division, addition, and subtraction) can be performed on two or more signals acquired at the same time. Another mathematical operation is taking the logarithm of the signal. This is useful for data compression where there is a very large range of signal level. Signal rectification is used to swing bipolar signals—signals that have both positive and negative levels—to levels that are all positive. Logic operations are used to indicate that the signal has achieved a yes/no, high/low, or on/off condition. This information is then used to trigger other signal processors to perform some function.

For example, I wanted to measure the heat content of expired respiratory gas. The heat content is proportional to the product of the volume of the gas and the gas temperature (water content of the expired gas is the proportionality factor). Since temperature changes continuously during expiration, heat content of a unit volume of expired gas is the product of instantaneous temperature and flow, and the total heat content during expiration is the integral of this product over time. We built a signal processor that multiplied expired temperature and flow rate and then integrated that product over time.

7

The Instrumentation Chain:
III. Display Devices, Recorders,
and Cables

The instrumentation chain has taken us to the point of actually observing the signal. Although the instruments used thus far are fairly standard and mandated by a narrow range of factors, there is a diversity of display devices and recorders whose selection is driven by a host of factors. These include not only the characteristics of the observed signal, but also the analysis that is planned for the observations. As an analogy, the stereo component system, to which we referred in chapters 5 and 6, includes instruments that are used for observation of the music signal. In fact, the whole point of the stereo system is to bring the music signal to the point where it can be observed.

The speakers and the audio meters of the stereo system are *display devices:* they convert the previously transduced, amplified, filtered, and processed signal from an electrical form to one our senses are capable of observing and interpreting. The audio meter is either a galvanometer or light display instrument that permits visual observation of the music signal. The speaker is a strain gauge transducer operated in reverse: electrical energy drives an electromagnet, which moves a diaphragm, which generates pressure waves of sound. This permits auditory observation of the music signal. This is also what instrumentation display devices do: they permit the temporary observation of a biologic signal as a visual or auditory display.

If a permanent record of sound wave signals is required, the tape deck of a stereo system is used: it captures the music on magnetic media and permits the signal to be retrieved and reviewed without recreating the original music signal. This is also what instrumentation recorders do: they permit the permanent recording of a biologic signal on paper or magnetic media. It can then be studied and analyzed multiple times without resorting to a recreation of the original signal.

WHAT YOU NEED TO KNOW

1. The capabilities of the display/recording device need to be matched to the requirements of the measuring environment, to the information content of the signal, and to the planned analysis of the signal. Sometimes more than one device is required to meet all these requirements. High cost is a major limitation.

2. Devices can be categorized by the frequency response of the information they can display, and the permanence and retrievability of the record they create.

3. Connectors and cables are mechanical links that are vital in the instrumentation chain. Their great promise is the ease and flexibility in the connections they can make between and within instruments. Their great failing is in the fragility of construction and the confusion in application.

Matching the Experimental Need to the Display/Recorder Device

You've got a high level signal output available from your amplifier and signal processor. Now what will you do? The observation must be changed back from its electrical energy form to one that is suitable for a human to understand. The exact device to be chosen depends on the properties of the signal you have observed, the environment in which you are making your measurements, and the short- and long-term plans you have with respect to the data analysis and archiving (Table 7–1).

TABLE 7–1.

Characteristics of Display Devices and Recorders*

TYPE	FREQUENCY RESPONSE	FORM OF DISPLAY	PERMANENT RECORD	COST/CHANNEL ($)
Light	DC to a few Hz†	Intensity, color, or pattern	No	10^1
Meter				
Analog	DC and very-low-frequency	Needle movement	No	10^2
Digital	DC	Digits	No	10^2
Audio	10^0–10^4 Hz	Pitch, intensity	No	10^2
Oscilloscope	DC–10^6 Hz	'x'–'y' light	Possible	10^3
Pen	DC–10^0 to 10^2 Hz	'x'-time tracing	Yes	10^2
Noncontact	DC-10^2 to 10^4 Hz	'x'-time tracing	Yes	10^3
Tape	DC-10^2 to 10^4 Hz	Playback through another display or recorder	Yes	10^3

*Frequency response and cost/channel are quoted as a power of 10. Actual values will vary, but usually will be within ±50% of this power of 10.
†Some light displays are limited not only by physical characteristics, but also by the limitations of the human eye to discern flicker.

Matching the Recording Needs to the Signal Properties

One of the major features we want our display/recorder device to have is the ability to present all the information content of the signal. As required of all instruments, we will select a device that has the appropriate bandwidth. There are limitations that impair the investigator's choice as to the type of display/recording and cost of the instrument in order to achieve a high-frequency response.

Matching the Recording Needs to the Environment

There are a host of considerations that are worth mentioning. These include some physical attributes of the recording device such as space, portability, power requirements, safety, and duration of recording capability. There are measurement attributes including the immediacy of displaying the observation, and the form in which the measurement is to be displayed. Consider some examples.

A very large tape recorder capable of storing multiple signals could well be appropriate for an experimental laboratory. But information stored on magnetic tape cannot be immediately viewed. In the clinical laboratory, there are valid needs for the real time (immediate) display of multiple channels of information that could dictate the choice of an oscilloscope display as well as a direct writing recorder. In the intensive care unit of a hospital, even the immediate availability of an oscilloscope display of information might be inadequate, and an auditory display (an alarm) may be used to provide supplemental information to the observer. If the signal to be observed comes from an ambulatory or remote source, we might consider a small portable device with low power consumption requirements and have to decrease the number of signal channels that can be recorded as well as the availability of immediate visual display of information.

Perhaps the major ergonomic consideration is cost. Display devices are inexpensive. However, many applications require a permanent record. Recording devices are by and large *the most expensive single instrument of the instrument chain.* Investigators commonly learn that all of their elaborate plans for data acquisition are frustrated because of their inability to obtain an inexpensive recording device.

Matching the Recording Needs to the Planned Analysis

The choice of a display/recording device is also importantly dependent on what type of analysis is planned for the data, and what degree of permanence of the recording is required. If a record is to be perused, measured, thought about, and shown to others, then it will need some form of permanent storage. If details of the record are to be reanalyzed, especially with the aid of additional instrumentation, then it may need to be recorded in a format that is suitable for further processing.

Types of Display and Recording Devices

There is a wide variety of display/recording devices, from the very simple forms of visual and auditory devices to sophisticated electromagnetic display and high-speed recording devices.

Visual Displays

The main advantages of simple visual display devices are their low cost and their ability to immediately communicate some information to the observer. Their disadvantages are the ephemeral nature of the communication (information cannot easily be saved), and their bandwidth, which is essentially DC. An important exception to the bandwidth limitation is the oscilloscope, which is discussed below.

Light Display.—This is the most primitive variety of visual display device. It conveys visual information by altering the intensity of a particular light, the number or position of multiple lights, or rarely by changing the flickering frequency of a light. For example, an engineer

I once worked with built a small and portable amplifier-display instrument that was used to detect tiny leakage currents from clinical instruments that could pose a shock hazard (see chapter 1). It has been accepted that a leakage current of less than 10 microamps is probably safe, whereas greater than 10 microamps is not. The test instrument lit a green light if the leakage current was less than 10 microamps *or* a red light if leakage current was 10 microamps or more. This is simple yes/no or on/off information that is useful.

Analog Meters (Galvanometers).—The leakage current testing device I mentioned above is only appropriate for a quick check of function, and is not useful as a certifying device where an actual quantitative measurement of leakage current is required; a device is needed that provides a quantitative readout, and that is what meters are capable of. An *analog meter* uses a galvanometer, which is a coil (inductor) wrapped around a magnet, which produces a circular deflection in proportion to the electrical energy of the input. The galvanometer swings a pointing device attached to it. The degree of deflection is quantitated by a calibrated scale toward which the pointer is directed.

Because the metering mechanism is a mechanical device that has a bandwidth that is essentially DC, the analog meter is most useful to display the constant or DC level of a signal. This is useful for raw signals that have a near DC frequency content, and for processed signals (such as the mean) that have a near DC frequency content. However, the human brain has an excellent capacity to remember short-term changes and trends. Analog meters, because their bandwidth is just slightly greater than DC, have the capacity to track small and slow changes. This trend information can sometimes be retained in the short-term memory of the observer's brain and proves to be of value.

The energy required to swing the needle of a galvanometer alone is small to moderate—energy requirements are much larger if the galvanometer drives a pen across a paper—and therefore these were the first devices used to quantitatively measure the output from electrodes and transducers without the assistance of amplification. This is of historical interest only, and to avoid loading down the signal source all modern galvanometers are linked to a power amplifier to increase the energy of low-level signals. Also, a prior stage of amplification is very important to assist in calibration and error correction (see below).

Some biologic measurements are made directly in voltage units, such as millivolts of bioelectricity. But many signals require that the observation be made in other biologic units such as *dimensions* of concentration, mass, flow, or pressure. In that situation, the scale of the meter has been calibrated by applying a standard biologic signal through the other parts of the instrumentation chain in order to yield a given electrical output. Usually the instrument manufacturer has performed the calibration and provided a scale in biologic dimensions. But some all-purpose or prototype metering devices reveal the true nature of the galvanometer, and require that the user apply the appropriate calibration.

Meters are subject to gross reading error, such as misinterpreting the printed number on the scale, and to fine reading error, such as parallax in lining up the pointer perpendicular to the scale. Meters are also fragile mechanical devices. They are easily ruined or uncalibrated by sudden, sustained, or large signals, and by mechanical trauma. All values out of range of the electrical capabilities of the galvanometer or the physical range of the scale will be clipped. If the scale is appropriately constructed, a maximum signal level should be distinguishable from a clipped level. Mechanical devices such as pointers may become stuck at the ends of the scale when an out-of-range condition occurs, and a further change of signal back into the operating range of the meter may not be shown—the pointer may stay "frozen."* Analog meters are especially prone to offset errors that involve the displacement of the pointer, and they should include some capability for adjustment. Analog meters are less subject to proportional errors; because it is very difficult to adjust a proportional error in a mechanical device, usually no adjustment capabilities have been provided in the meter itself. However, if driven by an amplifier, it is possible to use the adjustments of the amplifier to correct for proportional errors.

Digital Meters.—These are extremely valuable examples of meter devices. Digital meters convert an analog voltage input to a numeric output; that is, they are digital voltmeters. In fact, in our laboratory we use a DVM as an all-purpose instrument including troubleshooting and signal measurement. Again, as in the analog meter, the fundamental instrument design is to provide a display of the electrical energy input to the meter. It is only through calibration to a reference source that biologic units can be provided on the display. Digital displays provide exact values, which may give the user a false sense of security about the accuracy of the information displayed. In the intensive care unit or animal laboratory, a clotted arterial catheter may seal pressure within

---

*This was alleged to occur in the Three Mile Island nuclear power plant accident, where the detection of the flow of cooling water was misjudged because the pointer of an analog meter became stuck.

the tubing and yield a mean arterial pressure on the numeric display that appears quite normal, while cardiovascular collapse goes undetected!

Some of the mechanical reliability problems associated with analog meters are reduced with digital meters because there are no mechanical components. Both offset and proportional errors due to the meter are minimized. Recovery time after an out of range condition is less than a mechanical meter, but still not instantaneous. An input that has a very high energy level may result in damage. Burnout or failure of the leading edge digit (highest place holder) can be a problem, because digital display devices purposely "blank" (do not display a value for) these digits when they are not in use. Therefore, it would not be possible to distinguish normal from failed operation unless the observer inferred that the observed value was an order of magnitude different from the expected value, and confirmed this by another recording device. Digital meters have substantially decreased in price.

Audio (Sound) Displays

Audio displays are useful in certain circumstances as alarm devices—that is, devices that are either "on" or "off," and provide a warning that some signal level threshold has been achieved. All of us who carry those accursed message beepers are aware of the effectiveness of their "message alert" tones. Alarms during experimentation and in the clinical setting also serve a limited purpose. Varying the pitch and intensity of an audio display could provide additional information, and this is sometimes used for testing human audition. An important and useful application is that of Doppler ultrasound flowmetry. Variations in flow velocity are presented as variations in pitch of the audio display. However, apart from lovers and apart from the aliens and scientists in the sci-fi flick *Close Encounters of the Third Kind*, very few of us can understand and accept the use of these simple audio displays for the transmission of sophisticated data. Advanced computer hardware and software have made human voice synthesis possible, and I expect this to be introduced into instrumentation in selected circumstances.

Oscilloscopes

Apart from other visual display devices are oscilloscopes. These devices have the ability to display information in two dimensions as an 'x' and 'y' display. Usually, the format of display is signal level ('y' axis) vs. time ('x' axis). In order to present this type of format, the oscilloscope links the electrical signal input to a timing device that sweeps the display across a cathode ray tube (CRT). Usually, the sweep across the screen of an oscilloscope is done repetitively: as the tracing reaches the physical limits of the display area, it is returned to the beginning of the display area. Like the mechanical movement of the pointer of a galvanometer across a scale, the oscilloscope moves a stream of electrons across a fluorescent surface. *Unlike a galvanometer,* an oscilloscope is capable of very high frequency response (DC up to a megahertz or more)—well beyond the requirements for biologic signal response. They are the gold standard for the display of biologic signals.

Apart from cost (they are moderately expensive), the other major limitations are in regard to the duration of display (limited) and the permanence of recording (requires additional devices). Except where provision has been made for retaining an image on the CRT screen (storage oscilloscope), the image is not retained on the screen. The maximum duration of the signal that can be displayed is the width of the screen (which ranges from a few centimeters to a few dozen centimeters) divided by the speed of the trace across the screen (which ranges from 0.01 to 2.5 m/sec or faster); as the screen is retraced, the previous information is blanked. Even this limited duration depends on a special screen phosphor to maintain the persistence of the image.

Because of their unparalleled bandwidth for visual display, great lengths were taken in the not too distant past to record information permanently directly from oscilloscopes by taking pictures from the CRT screen on single frame and motion picture cameras. The wide bandwidth of advanced direct writing recorders has eliminated the need for such practice when biologic signals are recorded.

As we have indicated for other visual display devices, the deflection of the signal on the CRT screen requires calibration, that is, reference to a biologic source for proper dimension and scale. Because of their great utility in calibrating and monitoring the progress of measurement, and because they provide for the immediate display of information, they are very useful even when a more permanent method of recording is employed. Many commercially available instrument packages—generally the ones available for big bucks or used for clinical purposes—will include an oscilloscope.

Paper Writing Recorders

Paper writing recorders are also known as chart recorders or hard copy recorders, because signal storage is accomplished by writing with some medium on paper. The writing source characterizes these recorders by name: pen (thermal, ink, or pressure), light (visible or ultraviolet), electrostatic, thermal print head, and ink-jet recorders. The types of writing devices also characterize many aspects of recorder specification.

The writing concept of all of these recorders is to physically or electronically move the writing device along one axis of the paper, while pulling the paper perpendicularly (rarely, circularly) under the writing device at a calibrated speed. Because they are elaborate devices and because they require supporting instruments to drive the writing apparatus, their cost is considerably greater than simple display devices. These are the premier and standard devices for permanently recording signals.

Chart recorders have a limited high-frequency response, and therefore bandwidth specification is of great interest (Fig 7–1). The specification of the cutoff frequency for a recorder is typically given at the 95% level of amplitude of the passband. That is, the specification value is that when the recorded signal has decreased to 95% of the flat portion of the bandwidth. Note that this is different from the convention used to describe the cutoff frequency of other instruments such as filters and amplifiers. Their passband is demarcated by the cutoff frequency at which the output amplitude has decreased to 3 dB or 70.7% of the flat portion of the bandwidth.

Pen (Thermal, Ink, or Pressure) Writing Recorders.—These chart recorders will directly contact the paper and deposit ink, heat a thermally sensitive paper, or apply pressure to sensitive paper. Their writing mechanisms have been honed over many years, and they are widely and successfully used. There are some disadvantages to these recorders based on their mechanical components. The frequency response is limited because the information is written by a pen or stylus that is directed to the proper place on the paper by a mechanical device. It should also be noted that frequency response for many pen writing recorders decreases as pen excursion increases. Specifications for a pen writing recorder are usually given as "from 'x' to 'y' Hz at 1 cm of pen deflection." Since channel widths are usually more than 1 cm, and since the user attempts to maximize resolution of the signal by taking full advantage of channel width, high-frequency response at increased pen deflection may not extend to the limits suggested by the specifications.

The simplest and least expensive example of this type of recorder is a mechanism that uses a servomotor to drive a cable to which is attached an ink pen or cartridge. The pen is moved in proportion to the signal in one direction while a chart of paper is pulled at a known rate under the pen perpendicular to the axis of pen motion. The advan-

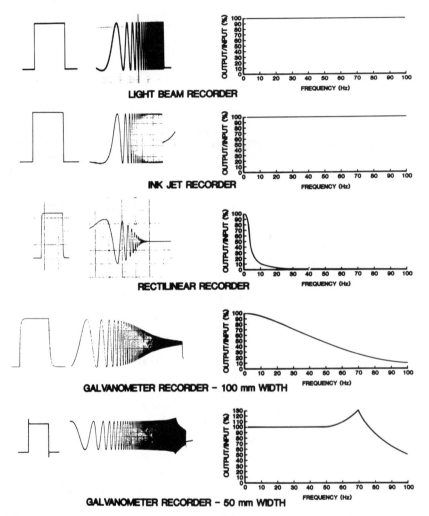

FIG 7–1.

Frequency response of recorders. Five different recorder tracings are shown from top to bottom: a photographic (ultraviolet) recorder, an ink-jet recorder, a rectilinear (servomotor-cable) recorder, a galvanometer recorder with a channel width of 50 mm, and a galvanometer recorder with a channel width of 100 mm. The frequency response of the recorders is evaluated with a square wave, shown at the far left, and with a frequency sweep (sine waves of increasing frequency) from 0 to 100 Hz generated by a function generator, shown next to the square wave. The typical frequency response diagram of the recorders, as determined from the frequency sweep (called a Bode plot), is shown on the right. The square wave demonstrates recorder response at the extremes of frequency: the upstroke and downstroke of the square wave evaluate the high-frequency response of the instrument tage of this system is that the writing characteristics are rectilinear—that is, the stylus is always perpendicular to the horizontal axis (which usually represents time) of the paper—and the pulley system is capable of moving large distances over the paper—that is, the channel width can be wide and resolution can be quite good. The disadvantages of the system are a limited frequency response with a typical bandwidth from DC to 3 to 5 Hz, and a limited ability to display more than one or two channels on the chart paper. Each pen requires a separate pulley that has to be physically offset from the other and, if the pens are to have a full range, must slide past one another. These recorders are principally used for low-frequency signals, such as plotting the output from the elution of a column of some biochemical process, or some physiologic process that has a bandwidth of low frequency, such as body temperature. They would not be useful for most physiologic events (see chapter 2).

A more sophisticated chart recorder will use a galvanometer to drive the weight of a pen or stylus, and has an improved high-frequency response compared to the pulley system. A typical frequency response specification could be a bandwidth from DC to 100 Hz, although many thermal and pressure recorders will be considerably below that high-frequency limit. As a rule of thumb, the high-frequency limit is inversely proportional to the length (and therefore the mass) of the pen. Why make the pen long? The range of motion—and therefore channel width and signal resolution—is proportional to the length of the stylus. Although many signal channels can be recorded on a single width of paper, each signal requires its own galvanometer and pen, and each channel must be physically separated from the others to avoid mechanical interference during pen movement. Channels are typically 40 to 50 mm wide, and the ability to record and resolve signals that have a wide range of levels can be a problem. Two solutions are suggested from chapter 6: (1) decrease the amplifier sensitivity that supplies signal to the recorder in order to reduce the level of the signal

---

and show an overshoot if there is resonance, and bowing or curving if there is attenuation. If neither is present, there is a sharp corner. The flat portion of the square wave shows the very-low-frequency response. Sagging or drooping would indicate a limit to low-frequency response (not as low as DC). The Bode plot shows more quantitative information about bandwidth. Note the frequencies at which resonance and attenuation occur for the rectilinear and pen writing recorders. Both the photographic and ink-jet recorder would also show limitation of high-frequency response if much higher frequencies were included in the evaluation. Compare this to the theoretical plot of frequency response of a second order system in chapter 3, Figure 3–2.

(but at the expense of decreasing resolution), or (2) use a logarithmic signal processor and record the signal as compressed data.

Many of these recorders are also prone to mechanical failure of the galvanometers and the pens. Pens on ink-writing recorders are especially prone to fouling,* while thermal recorder pens wear out. Because the pen swings on an arc circumscribed by the galvanometer, curvilinear recordings used to be the rule for this type of recorder (look at the motion of the pointer on a galvanometer). However, galvanometer-pen linkages are rectilinear on almost all modern chart recorders.

Noncontact Recorders.—These chart recorders accomplish their task without using a pen to directly contact the surface of the paper and, in some cases, without using a galvanometer. The photographic recorder (visible or ultraviolet light beam) is a very popular version of this concept. The position of an internal light source depends upon its deflection by a mirror attached to a galvanometer. Because signal change is recorded by deflecting a light beam instead of a pen onto photographically sensitive paper, there is a greatly improved frequency response of such recorders, and the bandwidth is usually from DC to beyond 5,000 Hz. The visible light beam recorder is an earlier version of this system. It required storing the exposed paper in a light-proof container and developing the paper in photographic chemicals in the dark after completing the data collection. This has now been abandoned, and modern recording papers develop as a wet or dry process as they are exposed to an ultraviolet beam and do not require postprocessing. The images are sharp and do not smear. There may be some limitation to very long-term preservation of the images. Because there are no pens or ink, and fewer mechanical parts, reliability is high and maintenance costs are moderate. However, this is offset by the very high cost of special sensitive paper.

The operation of the light beam offers the opportunity to multiplex many channels into the same display space. That is, because there is no mechanical interference with the operation of any signal channel (no pen has to "cross" in front of another) the potential display space for all channels is contiguous. The space allotted to a channel is adjustable at the discretion of the user. This has both beneficial and detrimental qualities. It is beneficial because any one channel can use almost the entire width of the paper and thereby improve resolution of the signal; also, signals can be overlapped for purposes of comparison or timing. It is detrimental because multiple signals that appear in the

---

*This sentence is dedicated to Tom Nusbickel.

same space and overlap can cause confusion. Of course, one could confine each signal to a separate display space, but the narrow width of the recording papers (in response to their expense) makes this somewhat undesirable. Devices that intermittently label the signals by channel designation and calibration on the paper during recording have been added in response to this limitation. There are two recently introduced recorders that provide an alternative to the expense of special recording paper required by the photographic recorder, but that retain many of the desirable features including bandwidth and signal multiplexing. They are the electrostatic recorder and the thermal print head recorder.

The electrostatic recorder is based on a combination of the light beam principle for high-frequency response, and the xerography principle for inexpensive recording. Because special recording paper is not used, very wide paper widths are available, which offers the opportunity to increase the resolution of the tracing. The electrostatic bonding of the carbon particles to the paper is permanent. The frequency response is comparable to the light beam recorder. The initial cost of this system is high.

The thermal print head recorder is based on the concept of a thermal strip or band that runs the whole width of the paper and that prints on thermal sensitive paper. This recorder has greatly increased capabilities of frequency response and reliability compared to the older thermal (pen and galvanometer) technology. The frequency response of this system is from DC to 500 Hz. Because the print head is a digital device, it is ideally suited for computer data acquisition systems (chapter 8), but can also be readily used with analog instrumentation. The initial cost of this system is competitive with other recorders.

Another recent alternative to pen writing or photographic recorders is the ink-jet recorder. These are galvanometric devices that direct a spray of electrostatically charged ink onto the paper. Because the ink-jet recorder eliminates the mass of the pen and its direct contact with the paper, high-frequency response is improved in comparison to pen writing recorders to about 500 Hz. But at high frequency there is air friction that distorts the ink spray pattern. Inexpensive chart paper can be used. However, channel width and reliability of ink delivery is limited by the mechanical aspects of the galvanometers.

Limitations of Chart Recorders.—All recorders have bandwidth limitation. As emphasized throughout this book, the frequency response of the instrument must meet or exceed the frequency content of the signal. To demonstrate this point, I recorded a signal on two of the recorders described previously: a pen galvanometer and a photographic recorder. The bandwidth of these two recorders shows that there will be visual differences in a recorded signal with frequencies above 50 Hz (see Fig 7–1). The signal I recorded is the great octave "C" of a clarinet, which has a fundamental frequency of about 65 Hz, and a frequency content that extends above 650 Hz (see chapter 2). Note the striking differences in the recordings made on these two instruments (Fig 7–2). The pen galvanometer shows the signal as a sinusoidal wave, whereas the photographic recorder captures all the nuances

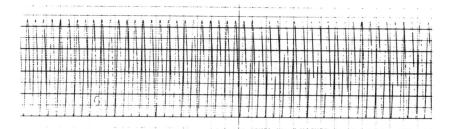

GALVANOMETER RECORDER

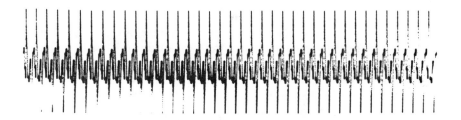

UV WRITING RECORDER

(f=65 Hz)

FIG 7–2.
Recorder with inadequate frequency response for the signal. The signal—the great octave "C" of a clarinet—was recorded on a galvanometer pen recorder *(top)* and a photographic recorder *(bottom).* The frequency content of this signal includes a fundamental of 65 Hz, but also a large number of harmonics such that high frequencies are present up to about 1 kHz. Note that in comparison to the high-frequency recording capability of the photographic recorder, the pen recorder is capable of recording the fundamental frequency of 65 Hz, but loses essentially all resolution of other frequencies in the signal.

of the other deflections that are truly present in the signal. This occurs because the pen galvanometer dampens or attenuates the amplitude of frequencies that are above a few dozen hertz, whereas the photographic recorder has a bandwidth that extends to a few thousand hertz. Translate this demonstration to your own requirements.

There are some other limitations to paper recording related to data analysis and archiving. Once written on paper, subsequent analysis of data is limited to what can be accomplished on a piece of paper with simple measuring tools. This includes the timing of events and the relationship of one event to another (in a multichannel recorder), and some painstaking efforts at precisely measuring signal level in the small space allotted for the recording. Another limitation is the great bulk and cost of recording paper that has to be recorded and stored in order to capture and preserve what can be only a small amount or short duration of signal. Witness the paper storage of a modern catheterization laboratory or especially a clinical electrophysiology laboratory, where the aphorism that there are "hours of boredom and moments of sheer terror" is exemplified by the large rolls of paper gathered in these studies. Hours of recordings are pored through to examine a few seconds', or sometimes a few milliseconds', worth of data. There is an alternative, or perhaps more appropriately a supplement, to the paper writing recorder—the magnetic tape recorder.

Magnetic Tape Recorders

A multichannel tape recorder capable of storing biologic signals is generally a bulky and expensive instrument. But, large numbers of signal channels and very long duration of events can be stored inexpensively and compactly on the medium of magnetic tape. Furthermore, because the signal is still in electromagnetic form, it can be recalled for analog and digital processing (see chapter 8) and recalled multiple times without having to repeat the data collection.

Now the bad news: in order to retrieve the data, the record has to be accessed serially. That is, in retrieving signals, the user will have to begin at the beginning of the tape and search the information stored on the tape in the order in which it was acquired. This search is usually performed by playback of the signals onto an oscilloscope. This laborious process can be reduced somewhat by careful record keeping during the experiment of the time at which a signal of interest occurred, the behavior of associated signals at the time of the event of interest, and value of the tape counter (a device that keeps track of how much tape has been moved). The tape playback is usually laborious and time consuming compared to a rapid visual scan by the observer of records made on a chart recorder. This is the current practice for clinical devices such as the 24 multihour ECG (Holter) tape monitor. A major advance in the analysis of electromagnetic tape has occurred by use of the computer. The computer can be programmed to recognize the characteristics of signals and to catalog events as a supplement to, or even in place of, human labor.

Because most clinical laboratory work plunges ahead with little time to review or ruminate, the review of data recorded on magnetic tape imposes an extra time-consuming step. In many research laboratory environments, the pace of work and the interest in further extracting data from analog signals is less frenetic, and this encourages the use of the magnetic tape recorder. In selected environments, digitizing data during the actual experiment and storing the data as digital rather than as analog signals on magnetic tape has become standard practice (see chapter 8). In this environment, a magnetic tape recorder will be used to store in detail part or all of the experiment. Simultaneously, for purposes of backup and early review of data, short periods of interest will be recorded on paper.

Connectors and Cables

Most instrument chains are linked together by cabling and connectors. Like the aphorism about a chain only as strong as its weakest link, so cabling and connectors are vital, yet cause problems.

Why Are Cables and Connectors Needed?

Instruments are a hierarchy of electrical and electronic parts. The instrument chain is a sum of these parts, and the parts need to communicate with each other. The parts themselves are divisible into smaller components, and the components need to communicate with each other. Many of the cables and connectors of instruments are "transparent" or concealed from observation because components are hidden within cases. But at each component, at each part, and at each instrument, there must be a port that provides communication to another component, part, instrument, or the outside world. The connector is that port, and the cable is one of the devices used to connect those ports.

Cables

These are the flexible wire links that transmit the signals or electrical power between connectors. Physically, cables are specified by the number of and size of wires or conductors they contain, by the geometrical arrangement of those conductors, and by the materials used in construction. Cables are used *for communication of signals, for transmission of electrical power, or for both.*

Power Cables (Cords).—These cables are used to carry electrical energy from a source of power (wall socket or power supply) to an instrument. Power cords that carry AC line voltage are usually a simple arrangement of three insulated conductors—hot, neutral, and ground—wrapped in a tough plastic or rubber sheath (Fig 7–3). In order to minimize a decrease in voltage due to the resistance of the conductors of the power cord, the size of the conductors is based on the expected current flow and the length of the cord: the larger the current flow and the longer the cable length, the larger the conductor (lower the wire gauge) size required. For example, a power cord of a few feet in length that had an expected current flow of a few amps would be constructed of 18-gauge conductors, while a cord that carried up to 15 amps would be constructed of 14-gauge conductors. Because power cords are expected to be somewhat flexible, their conductors will usually be multistranded, that is, they will be made of multiple fine copper wires twisted together to achieve the stated gauge size. The jacket or rubber sheath surrounding the conductors is specified according to the environment to which the cord is subjected. A hostile environment of chemicals, grease, high temperature, or direct sunlight will require a special jacket.

Power cords that link a power supply to an instrument may be similar to an AC power cord. Alternatively, power conductors may be included along with signal conductors as part of a multipurpose cable or umbilical cable. You've witnessed such cables rupturing away from a rocket during blastoff. Those umbilical cables may contain dozens or hundreds of conductors carrying power or signal. Multipurpose instrument cables also contain conductors for both power and signal. The cable from a strain gauge amplifier to a strain gauge transducer usually has conductors that carry electrical energy from the power supply of the amplifier to the transducer's Wheatstone bridge, as well as conductors for transmission of signal output from the bridge back to the amplifier.

Signal Cables.—These cables are used to carry signals between instruments, or within components of an instrument (Fig 7–4).

A major concern in the transmission of a signal by a cable is contamination of the signal by noise or interference in the environment, or conversely, contamination of the environment by the signal. In that regard, cables are selected by the noise or interference environment they will encounter. Especially subject to noise are cables that carry

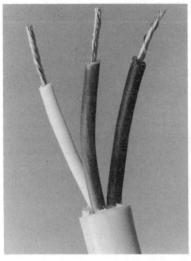
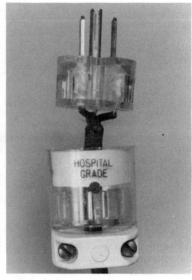

FIG 7–3.
Power cord and line plug. Standard components used to provide line power for instruments. *(Left)* three-wire power cord. The three conductors (hot, cold, and ground) are multiple strands of wire, each of which is covered by an insulative sheath. All three are bound together by another sheath. *(Right)* partially disassembled "hospital grade" plug. This plug is considerably different from that found on home appliances. The three conductors of the power cord are connected securely to the blades of the line plug as part of a separate platform. When fully assembled, this platform pushes back into and is secured as part of the case of the plug. Some "hospital grade" plugs are made of transparent material to facilitate visual inspection of the part of the power cord within the plug.

low-level signals (low energy, usually in the microvolt or millivolt range). The strength of the usual electromagnetic field surrounding a signal cable could swamp a low-level signal. The common mode rejection of a differential amplifier can handle much of the common mode interference that arrives with the signal. But, cables constructed for use with low-level signals are designed to minimize the effects of electromagnetic interference while the signal is within the cable. As important as it is to keep environmental interference out of a signal within a cable, it may also be important to keep a signal within a cable from passing interference to the environment. Noisy signals are generated from a variety of digital (computer) and radio frequency (TV, radio) sources.

Shielded cable is the standard cable for the transmission of low-level or inherently noisy signals. These signals can be either single ended or differential (see chapter 6). An example of a shielded cable is a coaxial cable, which consists of a central conductor concentrically surrounded by, but separated from, a shield. In a coaxial cable, a single-

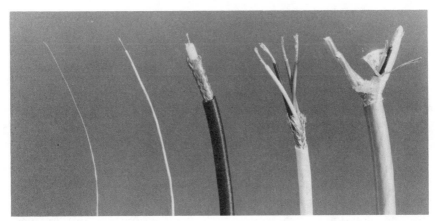

FIG 7–4.
Signal cables. Examples of simple and more complex signal cables are shown. *(Far left)* bare (no insulation) solid "hookup" wire. This is only used between components within a covered instrument to make connections between one point and another. *(Second from left)* insulated solid wire. May be used to connect electrical components within an instrument to prevent accidental contact with another wire or case, or may be used to transmit signals or low voltage power between instruments. *(Center)* coaxial cable, widely used with radio frequency (radio and TV) signals. The solid central wire is widely separated by a thick insulative foam from a coaxial braided wire sheath. The sheath surrounds the central conductor and prevents external noise from reaching the signal transmitted down the central conductor, and vice versa. *(Second from right)* multiconductor shielded cable. Extends the concept of the two cables immediately to its left. Multiple single conductors (four in this cable) that could carry signal or low-level power are insulated from each other and surrounded by a braid that separates the information in the cable from outside noise. *(Far right)* advanced multiconductor cable. This is a more advanced version of the cable next to it. It actually consists of three multiconductor cables, each with its own insulated conductors and shield, assembled together and surrounded by an aluminum foil shield. The shield is in continuity with the bare wire *(far right of picture)* that will connect to the ground pin of the connector.

ended signal is transmitted down the solid or stranded central copper conductor wire. Surrounding the central conductor, but separated from it by a concentric ring of insulation, is a wire meshwork or conducting foil that runs the entire length of the cable. This meshwork will be connected to ground, that is, it will contact the instrument cases (which have been connected to ground) at both ends of the instrument link. Any electromagnetic noise in the environment, or generated within the signal, will be picked up by the outer meshwork of the cable and passed to ground. If this interference comes from the environment, it will be picked up by the shield and passed to ground, while the signal within the central conductor will be protected. If this interference is part of the signal, it will be captured by the shield and passed to ground, while the environment will be protected. A variety of shielded cables exist for use when more than one central conductor is required.

High-level signals (high energy, usually in the volt range) are essentially not subject to the problems of environmental interference, because signal level is many times larger than the potential noise level that can be induced in the cable. Except in extremely noisy environments, high-level signals do not require shielded coaxial cables. Cables that transmit high-level signals use stranded or solid copper wire surrounded by insulation, which avoids grounding the signal to a metal object or to another wire. Two or more conductors may be contained within the same cable, and for protection will be surrounded by a jacket or sheath.

Power loss within a cable carrying a low-level signal is not a problem because current flow is vanishingly small. This is ensured by connecting a low-level signal source, such as a transducer output, to a very high input impedance instrument, such as an amplifier. The diameter of a conductor within a cable that carries a low-level signal can be very narrow (high-gauge number). Power loss within a cable carrying a high-level signal may be important when current flow is very large, such as the high power required to operate a chart recorder. To avoid power loss, conductor diameter is commensurately increased (smaller gauge number).

Connectors

A connector joins together, fastens, or unites an instrument to a cable or a cable to another cable. They are the ports or gateways through which either electrical power or signal is exchanged. A connector is a two-part device. The nomenclature for these two parts is "plug" and "jack or socket." Colloquially, the plug is called the male fitting because it consists of an extension or extrusion. The jack or socket is called the female fitting because it consists of an indentation or impression that admits the plug. This description is actually a useful shorthand for communicating which part of the connector to which one is referring. Unfortunately, it is only useful for simple connectors.

The two parts of a connector are meant to precisely fit together, which is one of the sources of their failings. Another failing of connectors is the difficulty in providing continuous shielding of low level or noisy signals.

Power connectors.—Power connectors complete the job of a power cord at either end of the connection: the power source or the instrument. The most familiar connector is that of the two or three blade plug of a 115 VAC power cord and its mating wall outlet or sockets (Figure 7–2). Most plugs are constructed to fit into the socket in but a single way; the ground blade and the slightly different sizes of the hot (smaller) and neutral (larger) blades insures this. Although many power cords disappear without a connector into the bowels of the instrument, some terminate in a socket which joins a plug mounted on the instrument case. This is a flexible arrangement which allows removal of the cord when not in use, and replacement when needed. Note that the plugs on the cord and on the case are never "live" or carrying power when they are exposed, i.e. when they are not connected to a socket or outlet. This is a safety practice invoked in all exposed connectors which carry electrical power which poses a shock hazard.

A wide variety of power connectors are used inside the case of an instrument or a housing. The simplest is the screw connector, in which the conductor of the cable will be made bare at the end of the cable and wrapped around a screw. Sometimes a lug or simple fitting is crimped or soldered onto the bare wire to provide strength. The metal screw will be threaded into a metal standard which will not only hold the screw but will also be connected to the power input side of the instrument. This type of connector is widely used for quick and non-critical applications. Most residential wall outlets and switch connections are of this type, as are many power connections within the case of an instrument. A recent variation of this quick type of power connector is the push connector, which anchors a bare solid wire by friction.

Because power and signal conductors are sometimes mixed in cables, connectors must follow suit. It would be unusual and dangerous to mix a high energy power conductor with a signal conductor. However, low energy power and signal conductors may be bundled together.

Signal Connectors.—These are the plugs and jacks that transmit a signal between an instrument and a cable or from one cable to another. There is an enormous variety of signal connectors (Fig 7–5). Within some rules of thumb, the choice of a particular type from this bewildering selection is based primarily on personal preference, and secondarily on the type of cable and the type of signal being connected.

Probably the most ubiquitous connector for signal transmission is the phone plug and jack, which is used to connect a cable that carries a high-level signal. The plug and jack are available in three sizes—subminiature, miniature, and standard (also called ¼")—and two standard styles—two conductor and three conductor, although a multiconductor style is available. The conductors on the plug are labeled from distal to proximal (cable) end as "tip," "ring," and "sleeve." Frequently, in a single-ended signal, the tip is connected to live signal and

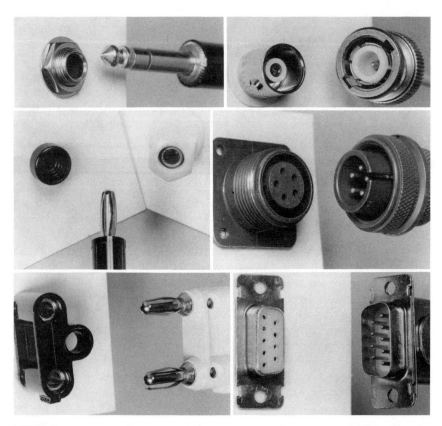

FIG 7–5.
Typical plugs and jacks (sockets) used in instruments. *(Top left)* three conductor, ¼" phone plug *(right)*. It will insert into a mating phone jack *(left)*, which has three discrete connectors to match those axially aligned on the jack. *(Center left)* banana plug *(bottom)*. This single conductor plug may insert into a banana jack *(left)* or a multiway binding post *(right)*. *(Bottom left)* dual banana jack *(right)*. It will insert into dual banana plug *(left)*. Because the plug and jack are symmetrical, they could be connected incorrectly. Note the flashing of plastic on the bottom of both the plug and jack that indicate the proper direction of mating. *(Top right)* BNC plug *(right)*. Central pin and outer sleeve match the jack *(left)*. A locking mechanism secures plug and jack together. *(Center right)* typical multipin connector used in analog instruments. An outer sleeve that has a "key" slot guides the correct connection of the five pins of the plug *(right)* into the holes of the jack *(left)*. *(Bottom right)* multipin connector ("D" connector) typically used in computers. The unequal lengths of the two sides of the connector guide the proper mating between the nine pins of the plug *(right)* and into the holes of the jack *(left)*.

the ring/sleeve connected to shield or ground. In a differential signal, the tip and ring may be the active or difference pair, and the sleeve is shield or ground. Unfortunately, there is no firm convention on this, and all who have encountered an instrument whose signal input/output connectors were unlabeled have spent many hours on a merry chase.

The banana plug and jack are another commonly encountered type of connector that is frequently used for a high-level signal. They come in a miniature and standard size. Each plug or jack is connected to but a single conductor. A variation on this is the dual banana plug, which molds two single banana plugs onto the same frame. The dual banana frame holds the two plugs on ¾″ centers that are meant to connect to banana jacks of the same center dimension. Because it may be important to identify the live signal vs. the shield or ground, one side of the dual banana is marked by a lug that is used to visually identify ground. However, this is a visual aid only, and doesn't guarantee that the user will connect the correct plug and jack together.

To obviate this problem, more sophisticated multiconnector plugs and jacks are always keyed. That is, all multiconnectors include a mechanical device, such as a slot or eccentric placement of blades, to ensure that plug and jack only can be connected in a single way. Multiconnectors may link a few or a large number of power conductors or signal conductors. Because their design allows an exact mating and low resistance pathway, they are frequently the choice for low-level signals. They can be linked by visually identifying the appropriate position of mating before insertion, or by gently rotating the plug until it readily slides together into the jack. Multiconnectors come in a bewildering variety of sizes, shapes, and number of conductors that can be accommodated. The user should remember that there is nothing special about these connectors: they were chosen by the instrument or connector manufacturer or instrumentation engineer because they met a handful of specifications that any one of a number of other connectors also could have met.

The BNC connector is a happy cross between a simple, yet secure, connector that is used for coaxial cable and therefore for low-level signals that use a single conductor with a shield or ground. Because of the coaxial arrangement and mechanical construction of the connector, I've never been able to discern which is plug and which is jack. However, the two parts are easily mated, and a partial turn locks them in a secure and low resistance connection.

Insulation displacement connectors (IDC or edge connectors) are those thin plated strips of metal that are lined up side-by-side at the edge of a circuit board. They are widely used inside of instruments to unite circuit boards. They are also used in instruments where external components are to be readily swapped in and out. The case of each component has an edge connector that provides a secure and precise multiple connection while in place, yet allows for the ready exchange with another component as desired.

The Instrumentation Chain:
IV. Computers

Computers have widespread application in the collection and management of data. Most laboratories, both clinical and research, are equipped with a variety of computers that serve multiple functions including word processing, data storage, statistical analysis, and instrumentation. It is the latter function that is the subject of this chapter.

The reader is warned that the following material in this chapter is technical and loaded with jargon. For those with a healthy skepticism about the merits of such material, you have my blessing to skip to the section entitled "Digital Analogs and Analog-to-Digital Conversion."

WHAT YOU NEED TO KNOW

1. Two elements compose the structure of a computer system: hardware and software. Hardware comprises all of the physical elements of the computer and includes components that are electronic, electromagnetic, and mechanical. Software is the set of instructions provided to the computer that regulate the hardware functions.

2. Digital computers process information in a discrete, nonanalog form. The fundamental unit of information is the "bit," which can be

thought of as a simple yes/no piece of information or as an on/off switch. It is rare for biologic signals, and transducers will have discrete states or values. More commonly, in order to make the transition from the analog form of information provided by transducers and amplifiers to the digital form of information (required by the computer), a special hardware/software device is required—the analog-to-digital converter.

3. When used as an instrument for signal measurement, the computer is typically at the end of the instrumentation chain, and therefore still requires much of the earlier hardware of the chain. Computers can serve as both observation and regulation instruments. In its former capacity, the computer serves mainly as a sophisticated instrument for recording and storing information. In its latter capacity, because of its decision-making capabilities (logic and artificial intelligence), the computer is especially adaptable to serve as an instrument that can control and regulate processes.

Classification

Digital computers are organized by their speed and sophistication of task performance: supercomputers, mainframes, minicomputers, and microcomputers or personal computers (Table 8–1). However, this classification has proven to be a relative one as the capabilities of each lower class have increased and the capabilities of the most powerful have achieved new limits.

Many computer users are unaware of the physical components and internal organization of the computer, but this may not limit their ability to use it effectively. For example, the user of large computers (mainframes) may conceive of the computer as a very large black box because there is a limited ability to access or control the internal structures. But the user of such a system may have substantial advantages by virtue of speed and simplicity of operation. On the other hand, the user of a microcomputer (small system and personal computer) tends to be more intimately aware of the physical components and system organization, but usually at the expense of spending additional time learning about and operating the computer. The descriptions below are structured for the microcomputer user, because it has become clear that these devices are the preferred form of computers used in instrumentation.

Hardware and Software

It is no accident that the design and structure of the computer is an anthropomorphism for the human brain. The computer system is

TABLE 8-1.
Classification of Computers*

TYPE	SPEED OF EXECUTION (OPERATIONS/SEC)	AMOUNT OF MEMORY (BYTES OF RAM)	BYTE LENGTH (BITS)	COMPLEXITY OF OPERATIONS	SPECIAL ENVIRONMENT	COST ($)
Supercomputer	10^7–10^9	10^8	64	Parallel	Yes	10^6
Mainframe	10^6–10^7	10^8	32	Fast serial	Yes	10^5
Minicomputer	10^5–10^6	10^7	16–32	Fast serial	Maybe	10^4
Microcomputer	10^3–10^5	10^6	8–16	Serial	No	10^3

*Speed of execution indicates the number of mathematical calculations (usually called floating point calculations) that can be performed in a second. Amount of memory is the amount of random access memory that can be addressed by the system. Byte length is the resolution of the system. The word *byte* is sometimes reserved for 8-bit resolution. Here it is used generically. Complexity of operations reflects the ability of the computer to do more than one task at the same time (parallel) or to do tasks in sequence (serial). Special environment indicates the required ambient conditions to operate the system including temperature, relative humidity, vibration, and other sources of radio frequency interference.

structured in very much the same way that the brain communicates and processes information. I will try to maintain this analogy in the descriptions that follow.

Hardware Analogy

The central processing unit or CPU (the brain) performs calculations, comparisons, and makes decisions based on information it receives and sends from input and output devices (sensory and communication organs) (Fig 8–1). Some of the computing and processing functions use short- and long-term electromagnetic storage devices (short- and long-term memory). The information is communicated to and from the various central and peripheral devices through bus structures and cables (central and peripheral nerves and ganglia).

CPU (Central Processing Unit).—The "brain" of the computer is an integrated series of electronic packages. A "microprocessor" is a type of CPU embodied in a single electronic package (chip or integrated circuit). The CPU is characterized by operating specifications. The *internal architecture* defines the size and the precision of the information by which the CPU receives information, performs calculations, and communicates results. This is measured in the number of "bits" with which the computer works. The larger the number of bits, the greater the precision of the operations of the computer. The *clock rate* defines the rapidity with which the CPU performs functions and cal-

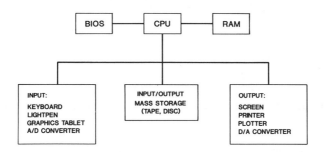

FIG 8–1.
Basic configuration of a computer system. The central processing unit (*CPU,* also called microprocessor in a microcomputer) operates under a minimum set of rules specified by the basic input/output structure *(BIOS).* The workspace for the CPU is random access memory *(RAM),* where additional instructions and data are stored and the results of intermediate operations are kept. The system receives and sends information to peripheral devices, some of which are suitable for sending information only *(INPUT),* some of which are suitable for receiving information only *(OUTPUT),* and some which both may send and receive *(INPUT/OUTPUT).*

culations. Every time the clock "ticks," the computer can perform another operation. The higher the clock rate, the more quickly a computer works. The *addressable memory* is the amount of workspace that the computer has access to in order to perform its functions. The greater the amount of memory, the larger is the workspace in which the computer can perform its jobs.

As an example, a widely used series of CPUs in small desktop computers—the 8088/8086 series—has the following specifications: its internal architecture is 16 bits, which means that it can resolve and calculate to one part in 65,536 (see below); it has a clock rate of 5 to 8 MHz; and it can directly address 1 megabyte (Mbyte) of memory. Another widely used series of CPUs—the 68000 series—has the following specifications: its internal architecture is 32 bits, which means that it can resolve and calculate to one part in 4.29×10^9; it has a clock rate of 8 to 12 MHz; and it can directly address 8 Mbyte of memory. These specifications for desktop computers have rapidly advanced in the past ten years, and current specifications are expected to be quaint ten years hence.

Input and Output Devices.—The sensory and communication devices of the computer are extremely important for providing information to and receiving information from the computer. Such devices may be strictly for *input or output,* and others may serve *both functions.*

A keyboard, card or tape reader, light pen, and graphics tablet allow the transfer of information such as letters, numbers, and symbols into the computer. A monitor (television) and printer allow the transfer of letters, numbers, and symbols out of the computer for the purpose of visual display. Disk drives, modems, and peripheral interface devices may receive, send, or store information depending on how they are configured. These *peripheral* devices greatly enhance the utility of the CPU; in fact, without them the CPU is virtually worthless, much as the chilling "locked-in" syndrome that can follow a neurologic catastrophe.*

Memory.—The CPU utilizes memory to store and recall operating instructions (the program), and as a workspace to save the intermediate results of computations. Memory can be broadly classified as either chip memory or non-chip (disk and tape) memory. Memory can be

---

*A rare and severe manifestation of some neurologic disease, such as stroke, is the virtual cutoff of the efferent output of the cerebral cortex from the rest of the body. Thus, although the brain can receive sensory input and is "thinking," it has extremely limited output—it is "locked in."

classified further as read-write or read-only, and volatile or nonvolatile.

Chip memory is contained in electronic packages that are directly accessible (addressable) by the CPU in a random manner; that is, the CPU can theoretically access any portion of memory, in any order, and at any time. Not surprisingly, this memory is called _random access memory_, or _RAM_. Convention dictates that the acronym RAM be used to refer only to read-write memory. Read-write memory is analogous to a chalkboard. One can write on a chalkboard in one area, read a note from another part, and perhaps erase and reuse still another area, all in random order.

Read-write chip memory may be volatile or nonvolatile. The terms _volatile_ and _nonvolatile_ refer to the relative permanence of the content of the memory. Thus, a volatile memory will lose its contents when power is removed, while a nonvolatile will retain them. Nonvolatile memory is typically considerably more expensive than volatile memory, and its operating speed may be slow. Nonvolatility is achieved by use of permanent magnetic memory; volatile memory can be made temporarily nonvolatile by providing backup power (a battery) when the primary power is removed. One type of inexpensive RAM in common use is called dynamic RAM, or DRAM. DRAM is so volatile that its contents must be restored or "refreshed" many times a second.

Read-only memory, or _ROM_, is nonvolatile, that is, the contents of the memory are retained when power is removed. Read-only memory may be supplied with permanent data, or may be user programmable ROM, or PROM. ROM is used in all computers to retain "start-up" instructions and programs that give the computer its personality, or basic input-output structure (BIOS). Additionally, specific dedicated computer applications such as those found in appliances, traffic controllers, and specific instruments usually have the entire program stored in ROM. RAM and ROM are usually placed in close proximity to the CPU, and are frequently housed in the same case.

Non-chip memory is used when massive amounts of nonvolatile memory are required. This mass storage memory may be housed within the same case as the CPU, or remote from it. This form of memory may be either read-write or read-only and can be characterized as either serial or random access.

With serial mass storage, data begin at the beginning and end at the end. The computer is required to search forward from the beginning of the storage media for the requested data. A seldom encountered form of serial storage, which saw extensive use as a storage medium in the early years of the computer age, was punched paper tape. This form of storage consisted of paper tape that could be punched with holes, the patterns of which could be read and interpreted as data.

Another type of mass storage read-write memory in wide use is magnetic tape in cassettes or on reels. The computer searches forward from the beginning of the tape for the requested data. New additional data are appended to the end of the existing data on the tape. Magnetic storage is compact, inexpensive, readily catalogued, easily retrieved, and resistant to deterioration—witness the ability of the IRS to maintain track of your income tax files.

Random access mass storage memory most commonly takes the form of magnetic disks. These disks either may be removable or fixed in the disk drive and can be further classified as being "floppy" versus "hard." These adjectives refer to the physical characteristics of the storage medium; an 8-in floppy disk will flop if held by a corner and shaken, a 20-megabyte hard disk cartridge won't. Technological developments, such as the appearance on the market of a 3½" floppy disk in a hard shell (that won't flop) have blurred these distinctions. Floppy disk storage systems may use either 8, 5, or 3½" format disks, and have capacities of up to 1.2 megabytes at present. Their advantage lies in low cost, removability, and portability. Nonremovable or fixed hard disk storage systems can store from 5 to well over 2,500 megabytes. Their advantage lies in high storage capacity and speed of data transfer. The speed of data transfer increases considerably as one goes from tape to floppy disk to hard disk. For example, a hard disk transfers data approximately five to ten times faster than a floppy disk. In general, high speed and random access are more expensive than low speed and serial access.

The most recently introduced mass storage technology is that of laser disks. These have rapidly evolved from read-only mass storage memory (called compact disk, or CD ROM), to write once and read mainly (WORM) read-write mass storage. Currently, read-write erasable disks with optical technology are under development. Their advantage lies in very high storage capability. While speed of transfer is better than most mass storage media, it is not as fast as that of a high-performance disc.

Bus or Communication Structures.—The CPU requires connections (bus or interface) to its input/output devices and memory. In simplest form, a bus is a mechanical device capable of making multiple connections for the transfer of electrical or electronic signals. The connections are organized in a manner that is standard for that particular bus. Each computer system will have a bus structure to make these connections. This "internal" bus structure varies with the computer and presents a myriad of compatibility problems. An exception to this is, for example, the S-100 (IEEE-696) bus structure, which represents an attempt by the computer industry to set standards for the internal connection structure of certain microcomputers.

For a variety of reasons, standardized bus structures that communicate with "external" devices such as printers and modems have received greater acceptance by computer manufacturers. In addition to the mechanical aspects of these bus structures, such as the type and placement of the pins of their electrical connectors, the bus may have additional specifications such as the speed of information transfer, the size and sequence of information transfer, and the voltage and electronic characteristics. As industry standards are developed, computer manufacturers may adopt none, some, or all of these standards for their computers.

The RS-232 (serial) bus structure is an example of a standard interface that is commonly used for modem and for printer communication. The Centronics (parallel) interface is commonly used for printer communication. The IEEE-488 bus or interface structure (also called the GPIB, or general purpose interface bus) is a parallel bus sometimes used for disk drives, printers, and many laboratory and scientific instruments. Manufacturers and professional organizations are currently developing new standards that would be applicable to many medical and scientific instruments.

Software Analogy
We are all born with a limited but useful set of nurturing brain instructions. These instructions fall into two categories: instructions that allow us to carry out fundamental brain functions (innate behavior), and instructions for basic learning skills that allow us to increase the instruction set of the brain and therefore emit new behavior (learned behavior). Additional complex learning greatly enhances the power of the brain. The full extent of this starting set of instructions is sometimes not discovered until additional learning occurs that relies partly on the nurturing brain instructions. Analogously, the CPU is usually provided with some minimum instruction set that governs its organization and communications behavior and provides the means by which additional sets of instructions (program) can be entered into the computer—the BIOS.

BIOS.—The basic input/output structure—BIOS—is a set of instructions for the operation of the CPU's organizational, computational, and logic behavior. The program is stored in nonvolatile memory (usually ROM) and accessed by the CPU at the time of power-on. This set of instructions could be the entire program for the operation of the CPU if it were dedicated to a specific task. This is very useful for CPUs with a defined purpose. Such CPU-ROM combinations are widely used as part of other instruments such as signal processors or recorders. These instruments are assigned fixed and repetitive tasks without the requirement for programming modification.

However, if the intent is to use the CPU for a variable series of tasks, including tasks that may evolve or be added, then an additional function of the ROM will include a method for inserting new instructions into the CPU in order to alter its behavior. This is called programming.

Programs.—The set of instructions (the code) provided to the computer to direct its function is called a program. The route of entry of this program into the computer may be by keyboard, if the program is being created for the first time. The program may be recalled from a storage device (usually a disk) if it has been previously created. A program may be entered from a PROM, if a suitable interface has been provided.

The instructions will have to be in a language the CPU understands. This ultimate or lowest-level language is called machine language, and is the unique instruction set for a particular CPU. It consists of 1's and 0's that compose the information stored in the bits, which are then organized into bytes, which the computer translates into action. However, there are additional languages that can be used to program the computer (Fig 8–2).

Shortly after the introduction of computers, problems with programming in machine language were recognized. First, machine language was alien to the language skills of humans programming the computer. Second, the coding for machine language was slow and tedious, because each step of microprocessor function required specification—each bit had to be programmed. Third machine language was CPU specific and therefore programs were not transportable to a new CPU.

In order to obviate these shortcomings, "higher-level" computer languages were created. For a language to be useful, it has to (1) reduce the laborious programming tasks of moving bits of information around one step at a time, (2) have a syntax that is readable by the programmer and anyone else trying to understand the code, and (3) if

BASIC

x=2+2
PRINT x

FORTH

2 2 + .

FIG 8–2.

Examples from four different computer programming languages. In each, the same application is addressed: the computer is to add together "2 + 2" and then print the results on a printer. While the instructions written in Basic are most intuitive, there are advantages to compactness, speed of operation, and ease of building a complex instruction set in the other languages.

ASSEMBLY (8088 CPU)

MOV AX, 2
ADD AX, 2
OUT SC, AX

"C"

PRINTf("%d", (2 +2))

feasible, should be transportable between CPUs. In order for the CPU to understand the programming instructions in these languages, an editor-compiler-linker must be available for the computer to convert the code back into machine language. In the end it is the machine language that the computer understands.

Assembly language goes part way toward fulfilling the requirements of a high-level language. It has some syntactical foundation (short mnemonic codes such as "add" are used as programming instructions) and it works at a higher level of organization than machine language. Additionally it is applicable within a family of closely related microprocessors, but cannot be transported to another series of microprocessors, since each family requires a unique assembly language.

A number of languages have been developed that fullfill all three of the above-mentioned criteria to some degree, such as Fortran, Basic, Cobol, Pascal, Forth, and C. The proliferation of languages reflects not only improvement in writing languages with improved syntax as well as improved speed and power of the compilers,* but also reflects the concept that some languages tend to perform some programming aspects better than others.

Digital Signals and Analog-to-Digital Conversion

Digital computers work with discrete, that is, noncontinuous information. This occurs because the fundamental unit of calculation in the computer is the bit (contraction of binary digit), which can either be a 1 or a 0. Analogously, one can think of this basic unit as an on/off switch or a yes/no answer. The math structure organized to this bit pattern is log to the base "x." The "x" is usually 2, hence the name binary numbers, but may be 8, 16, or any other number. It is also convenient to think of a bit as a letter of the alphabet. We can't do very much with individual letters until we organize them into larger strings called words. This is also what the computer does with its bits. The addition of successive bits to form larger units (called bytes or words, depending on the number of bits) allows very large and very small numbers and simple and more complex information to be represented in the computer.

Digital Signals and Computers

Because digital computers use only discrete signals, we are confronted with a problem for the use of computers as instruments. To our perception and measurement most biologic signals are nondiscrete and continuous, that is, analog. There are some exceptions to this. For example, "handedness," that is, the ability and preference to use the right or left hand in preference to the other, is inherently a yes/no or 1/0 (digital signal). Also, neurochemical transmission is the release of quantized or packeted neurotransmitters with discrete properties. However, these are the exception.

Almost all the transducers, amplifiers, filters, signal conditioners, display devices, and recorders and storage devices we have discussed in previous chapters communicate in analog signals. At present, none of these devices can communicate *directly* with a digital computer.

---

*The efficiency and speed of a program written in one of these languages depends on both the skill of the programmer in writing a program in that language, and the ability of the compiler to translate that program into an efficient and compact set of machine language instructions. Bear in mind that the CPU is capable of executing only machine language instructions.

Therefore, an additional device is required to perform this conversion—the analog-to-digital converter (A/D converter, Fig 8–3).

The A/D Converter

Many of the same specifications we described earlier in this book for analog instrumentation are also suitable for use with digital instrumentation, and the reader is advised to review chapter 3.

Concept of Digitization.—An A/D converter samples a continuous (analog) voltage signal and converts the signal level to a discrete voltage value. The voltage level is then translated into a numerical value called an A/D unit, which the computer can then handle as it would any discrete numerical value. Sampling of the analog signal may occur once or, more commonly, serially (Table 8–2). This concept of sampling is analogous to capturing a moment out of a continuous event by taking a snapshot and freezing the action.

Resolution of Sample.—The analog to digital converter resolves a signal based on the number of bits used for a sample, typically 8, 10, 12, 14, or 16 bits. For example, a resolution of 10 bits means that the A/D converter is capable of resolving the analog signal to 1 part in 2^{10}, or 1/1,024. Thus, if the voltage range (the range of the input signal that can be digitized by the device without clipping) of the A/D converter were 0 to $+10$ volts, a 10-bit A/D converter could resolve the signal to 10 volts/1,024 = 9.77 mV. If this same device had an input range of ± 1.25 volts, it would be capable of resolving 2.5 volts/1024 = 2.44 mV.

Precision and Accuracy.—It is important to understand the approximations that occur during digitization of an analog signal. They are of two types: (1) an approximation of the value of a signal that is

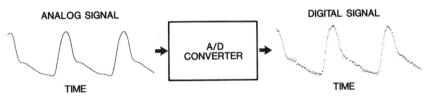

ANALOG SIGNAL   DIGITAL SIGNAL

A/D CONVERTER

TIME   TIME

FIG 8–3.
Digitization of analog data. The analog-to-digital converter *(A/D converter)* converts a continuous waveform into a series of discrete values. While the result is not as cosmetically pleasing as the original, it is the only method a computer has for dealing with information. Once converted, the power and sophistication of the computer can be applied to the data.

TABLE 8–2.
Digital Samples of Arterial Pressure Over One Cardiac Cycle*

SAMPLE NO.	DIGITAL VALUE (A/D UNITS)	PRESSURE, MM HG	SAMPLE NO.	DIGITAL VALUE (A/D UNITS)	PRESSURE, MM HG
. . .	. . .	. . .	432	2479	82.1
. . .	. . .	. . .	433	2474	81.2
407	2393	66.0	434	2469	80.3
408	2390	65.5	435	2463	79.1
409	2387	64.9	436	2458	78.2
410	2384	64.4	437	2453	77.3
411	2378	63.2	438	2449	76.5
412	2376	62.9	439	2447	76.1
413	2377	63.0	440	2445	75.8
414	2384	64.4	441	2442	75.2
415	2404	68.1	442	2439	74.6
416	2434	73.7	443	2435	76.1
417	2475	81.4	444	2432	73.3
418	2513	88.5	445	2431	73.2
419	2543	94.1	446	2427	72.4
420	2567	98.6	447	2424	71.8
421	2582	101.4	448	2421	71.3
422	2596	104.0	449	2418	70.7
423	2605	105.7	450	2416	70.3
424	2605	105.7	451	2412	69.6
425	2603	105.3	452	2409	69.0
426	2587	102.3	453	2407	68.7
427	2570	99.2	454	2403	67.9
428	2549	95.2	455	2401	67.5
429	2521	90.0	456	2396	66.6
430	2500	86.1	. . .	. . .	. . .
431	2485	83.3	. . .	. . .	. . .

*Conversion rate, 75 samples per second.

the precision and accuracy of the sample (described here); and (2) an approximation of its frequency content or bandwidth (described below).

An analog signal can assume any value, but a digitized signal can only assume discrete values equal to the range of the input divided by the resolution of the byte size. For example, suppose we use an A/D converter with a range of ± 10 V and an A/D device that has an internal architecture that specifies a byte as 12 bits. The signal resolving power with these specifications will be 20 V/4,096, which is about 4.9 mV, which is the value represented by a stored value of "yes," "on," or "1" in one bit. The typical specification for precision and accuracy of an

A/D converter is ±1 bit. This means that two values of the signal that are less than 4.9 mV apart (±50% of a 4.9 mV range of voltage) will not be resolved as different values.

Once the biologic and the voltage signal range are known, then one can judge the effect of digitization on precision and accuracy. For example, the typical output of an (unamplified) thermocouple is about 1 mV/°C. If we digitize this signal with the above specifications, we would have a precision and accuracy of about ±2.5°C. That might be just fine for monitoring the temperature of a blast furnace, but probably wouldn't be good enough for a biologic experiment with a temperature range of 20 to 40°C. In this situation, one could amplify the thermocouple output with a gain of ×250 before digitization to achieve a precision and accuracy of ±0.01°C. This suggests that the experimenter must know a considerable amount about the signal to be digitized as well as the expectations of the level of important changes of signal.

Frequency Response.—A second approximation in the use of digitizing instruments occurs because of the discrete sampling interval of the A/D converter. We have previously used the *Fourier theorem* to understand and specify the frequency content of a signal, and therefore, the specifications of the instruments that are to observe that signal. The Fourier theorem states that a periodic signal can be considered as the sum of an infinite series of sine waves of different frequencies. In practice, no more than a few dozen of these sine waves are needed to characterize the vast majority of the information contained in most biologic signals. But there is another theorem that determines the bandwidth of digitized signals.

The *sampling (Nyquist) theorem* states that it is necessary to sample data at twice the rate of the highest frequency that is present in the signal. In terms of the Fourier or spectral analysis, the highest frequency that can be represented from digitized data is one half of the sampling rate. For example, in order to reproduce the bandwidth of a signal with a frequency content of up to 20 Hz, one would have to—according to the Nyquist theorem—digitize at a sampling rate of at least 40 samples per second. If the bandwidth of the digitized signal includes higher frequencies than can be resolved by the sampling rate (i.e., frequencies more than one half of the sampling rate), the result will be an *aliasing* of the observed signal.

Aliasing is a type of sampling error that occurs when the sampling rate is too low. The result of this error is that the information of frequencies higher than the resolving power of the sampling rate actually appear mixed in with the lower frequencies, and this results in a distortion of the observed signal. The reader will recognize aliasing as a sampling limitation from everyday life, such as the appearance of a spoked wheel that appears to be standing still, or lazily spinning backwards or forwards during motion picture replay. This occurs because a motion picture is a series of still frames that typically "samples" the field of view at 24 frames per second. If the rotation of a spoke around the wheel between frames (samples) is $\frac{1}{n} \times 360^0$ (where n is the number of spokes in the wheel), the spokes will be in an identical position at the time of frame exposure, and this gives the appearance of no wheel motion. Slightly more or less angular motion between frame exposures produces the appearance of lazy forward or backward motion of the wheel. What we observe when the still frames are replayed is the bandwidth limitation of the sampled data mixed with the information of the higher frequencies of the actual bandwidth.

Therefore, similar to the knowledge of frequency content of the signal in order to use analog instruments (chapter 2), the experimenter must know the frequency content of the signal in order to set an appropriate A/D sampling rate for computer instruments. High-frequency components that are present in the signal, whether they are part of the true biologic signal or introduced through error and interference, can foul the information obtained by digital acquisition. Because of these concerns, which can introduce serious aliasing error, two steps are taken to ensure that the sampling rate is appropriate to capture the frequency content of interest. First, signals to be digitized are passed through a low-pass filter prior to digitization in order to remove high frequencies that are not important to the bandwidth of the signal. Second, sampling rate is increased beyond that required by the Nyquist theorem, usually by a factor of two.

Multiplexing Multiple Signals.—An A/D converter is only capable of quantizing a single signal at a time; thus, to observe multiple signals, the A/D converter input is switched between signals, sampling and converting each in succession. This process of switching between signals is called *multiplexing*. Typical multiplexed A/D converters may have 8, 16, 32, 64, or as many as 128 signal channels, depending on the computer and the application.

Speed of Digitization.—The speed with which the A/D converter can acquire the digital representation of one analog signal sample is called A/D conversion time. The conversion time alone, however, does not describe the dynamic characteristics of the conversion process. That specification is A/D throughout to memory, and includes the time for the multiplexer to "settle" on a channel (that is, provide a true representation of the analog signal), actual A/D conversion time, and the time required to transfer the binary value to the computer's memory. The difference between these two specifications can be large. A perusal of the data sheet of one manufacturer's A/D converter illustrates this difference. The A/D conversion time is specified as 25 microseconds, implying a sample rate of 40,000 samples/sec. However the A/D throughput to memory is 13,300 samples/sec, three times slower.*

Throughput.—When determining sample rates, it is important to understand that the actual sample rate per channel is the figure of importance. This is determined by dividing the total sample rate by the number of channels being sampled. If the total *throughput* were 10,000 samples per second, and seven channels were being sampled, then the sample rate per channel would be 10,000/7 = 1,428 samples/second/ channel. Likewise, if only one channel were being sampled, the sample rate per channel would be 10,000/1 or 10,000 samples per second. To obtain 1,000 samples/sec of 64 channels of data (for example, during heart electropotential mapping) would require an A/D converter with a throughput of 64 × 1,000 = 64,000 samples/sec. It is possible that the total requirements for digitization exceeds the specification for A/D converter throughput. In that case, two alternatives may be considered. Either reduce the total number of samples/second that are being digitized, or record the analog signals on magnetic tape and play the tape back at reduced speed while digitizing the prerecorded signals.

Computers as Instruments

The ability of a computer to gather and store information allows this device to be used as an observation and communication instrument. Because of its prodigious calculating abilities, the computer can also be used for data analysis. An additional, more powerful feature of the computer is its ability to apply decision-making to the input and to provide an output for the purpose of controlling a process that allows this device to be used as a regulation instrument.

---

*When referring to A/D sampling rates, the terms "samples/sec" and "Hz" are commonly used interchangeably. This is not correct and introduces confusion because it appears as if the sampling rate is synonymous with the frequency content of the data to be sampled (which is correctly stated in dimensions of "Hz").

Observation Instrument

When placed at the end of the instrument chain, a computer can serve as a display and recording device. These possibilities offer only marginal benefits compared to analog instrumentation. What is of major benefit is the ease of data archiving and data analysis that follows the recording of digital information.

The Data Logger.—The simplest form of a computer observation instrument is the data logger. The data logger consists of input and output ports, an analog to digital converter (if required), a microprocessor, a set of instructions (contained in the BIOS-ROM) and memory storage capability (contained in RAM). Its function is to store signal levels in digital memory, and to be able to retrieve those digital levels. Data loggers are frequently small, portable battery-operated instruments that are intended for data collection in remote or inhospitable conditions. Limitations of weight, size, and electrical power size may limit the amount of RAM and therefore the amount of data that can be stored. To overcome this handicap, data loggers frequently use data compression techniques such as intermittent data sampling or averaging. In that circumstance, the only data that are stored is the spot sample or the average value. Therefore, raw data are not available and the user must assume that the reduced data are representative of the whole data set.

Computer Systems.—At a more sophisticated level of observation, the computer instrument will have expanded programmability, RAM, and input/output devices. Data received as input into a digital computer following A/D conversion will be stored temporarily in RAM memory. From RAM memory, further decisions about data management are made. For example, it is frequently desirable to display data as they are acquired from A/D conversion. With very high-speed graphics capabilities, it is possible for the computer to display the digitized input signal on a monitor as a graph of data value against time (or possibly another dimension) almost simultaneously with its acquisition—in "real time". It may be appropriate to write the data from RAM to a nonvolatile form of memory, such as a magnetic disk, and to defer the display of data until a later time.

Data Storage and Analysis.—The greatest utility of the computer as an observation instrument can be appreciated after data acquisition. Through the use of storage devices, such as magnetic disks, the experimenter can recall and reanalyze data repeatedly. In contrast, a well-thumbed roll of recorder paper quickly loses its practical and aesthetic appeal. This recall ability offers the opportunity to ask new and additional questions of the data. Stored data can be displayed by computer monitors, printers, and plotters. Such graphic displays typically will be digital, that is, they will be shown as the characteristic discrete values acquired by the computer.

Another powerful feature of digital acquisition is the possibilities inherent in data analysis. The data values that exist in digital memory are in the form of numbers that, when provided with calibration, become dimensioned numbers. The full numerical analysis capabilities of the computer can be turned loose onto crunching these numbers. Many of the most powerful functions are mathematical functions, which analog signal processing emulates less successfully than digital signal processing: averaging, determining minima and maxima, integrating, differentiating, and filtering. The last function is particularly worth mentioning because it demonstrates the power of digital analysis.

As shown in chapter 7, filtering is an abstract concept that takes concrete form as analog filters are built from hardware components—usually electronic components. There are limitations to the performance of the hardware such that ideal filter specifications cannot be met. For example, there is frequently not a sharp roll-off between the pass band of the filter and the corner of the filter. Or there are limitations in designing filters with steep filtering slope. Many such limitations are obviated by digital filtering.

Numerical analysis includes statistical analysis. Once collected into a file, these data become the input for programs that provide statistical analysis. Although we have eschewed the use of mainframe computers as instruments, their power is a major advantage when it comes to data crunching and statistical analysis. It is quite common to collect the data on a small computer that serves as the instrument, and then to pass the data onto the mainframe for analysis. For example, large statistical packages such as "Statistical Analysis Systems" (SAS), "Biomedical Data Processing" (BMDP), and "Statistical Package for the Social Sciences" (SPSS) are now widely used on mainframe computers. Some of these programs have recently been adapted for microcomputers. Because of the ready availability of computer-based statistical packages, and the widespread appreciation of the importance of the application of appropriate and detailed statistical testing, most refereed journals now insist on this detailed analysis.

An Example—Spectral Analysis of Music.—In chapter 2, I showed you the Fourier analysis of a musical note from four different instruments. This was performed by the principles of the computer as an observation instrument.

The signal source was my child's music synthesizer, which itself is a computer with a D/A converter that provides an analog signal of the music. I decided to acquire a "C" note, and looked up its frequency characteristics. A "C" two octaves below middle "C" has a fundamental frequency of about 65 Hz. Because of my prior knowledge of the overtones present in musical notes ("Grandmother" principle), I wanted the frequency spectrum to include up to ten harmonics, which would be a bandwidth up to 650 Hz (ten times the fundamental frequency). According to the Nyquist theorem, this would require a sampling rate of 1,300 samples/sec. In practice, even a higher sampling rate is advisable. The output port of the music synthesizer (in this situation, acting as the signal source and transducer) was passed through a low-pass filter and then into an A/D converter.

A program was written that included code in "C" and assembly language and that instructed our microcomputer to control the A/D converter and to acquire the digitized data into memory. The CPU was instructed to write the acquired digital data into RAM temporarily, then display the digitized data on the computer monitor. The program also instructed the CPU to print a graphical display of the data onto a printer. Figure 2–7 (chapter 2) is a series of photographs made from the printed display. For permanent storage, the data were written on a hard disk. The data were analyzed after storage by recalling the data into RAM. The analysis part of the program included the instructions for the equations required for calculation of the Fourier spectrum. The output of amplitude and phase angle from the Fourier analysis were printed, and we translated those numbers into the bar graphs that appear in the Figure alongside the waveforms.

An Example—Analysis of Hemodynamic Data.—The microcomputer system also can be used for other types of signal processing. Multiple channels of data can be acquired and analyzed. In the top panel of the accompanying figure (Fig 8–4), I show the digitized waveforms of the electrocardiogram, the left ventricular pressure as well as the arterial pressure of an anesthetized rat. Two additional panels are shown.

In the middle panel, a display of some signal processing performed by the program on all three signals is displayed. The computer has detected and automatically marked the peak of the "R" wave of the

Record 07 of r43i-1 Recorded 06-21-85 10:06:28

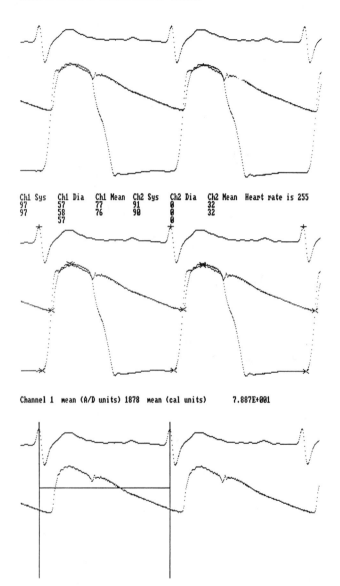

Ch1 Sys Ch1 Dia Ch1 Mean Ch2 Sys Ch2 Dia Ch2 Mean Heart rate is 255
97   57   77   91   0   32
97   58   76   90   0   32
         57   0

Channel 1 mean (A/D units) 1878 mean (cal units)   7.887E+001

FIG 8–4.

Examples from a microcomputer data acquisition and analysis system. In the top panel, the computer has digitized three analog signals, stored the data in RAM, then presented the data (in this case, printed it on a printer). The bottom two panels show various types of computer analysis performed on the signal, and further explained in the text.

electrocardiogram. By detecting this peak, the time between two successive peaks can be determined that is the period of the heartbeat, or its inverse, the heart rate. Similarly, the computer has detected and automatically marked the peak systolic pressures and the end diastolic pressures of the arterial pressure and the left ventricular pressure. The type of programming required for this analysis is more sophisticated than simply translating exact equations into program instructions, and is the type of analysis at which the computer excels. It is done by programming groups of instructions called algorithms. In this example, we use a set of rules based on timing relationships and relative and absolute minimum and maximum levels of the signal. These algorithms are, to some extent, based on heuristics or rules of thumb that we would use ourselves to analyze the data manually. Analog signal processors may also be able to do the same; but the more complex the rules and relationships, the more likely is digital analysis to be better than analog analysis.

In the bottom panel, a digital display of the arterial pressure and its mean level is shown. Determination of the average of a signal is a traditional type of analysis that could be performed by either analog or digital signal processing. In the microcomputer analysis, the program for the calculation of the average value of a signal is straightforward. It is based on a simple equation for summing the discrete levels of the signal over the period of the signal, and dividing by the number of levels that were summed (a correction, called the trapezoid rule, is made for the first and last levels of the signal). All of the types of signal conditioning mentioned in chapter 6—amplification, filtering, and signal processing—can be performed by the microcomputer on digitized signals.

Regulation Instrument

Computers have the ability to apply not only mathematical computations to data, but also logical testing. These two elements can be joined together in a part of a program called an *algorithm* for purposes of decision making. One of the outcomes of decision making could be the control of an output signal from the computer for the purpose of controlling a process.

Digital to Analog Conversion.   Let's face it, quantum mechanics aside, our perception of the world is still largely analog. However, the computational and logical processing performed by a computer is digital. We would like to take advantage of the powerful computational and logical capabilities of the computer for use in the real world. That's what happens when you retrieve, analyze, and interpret digital data. But it would be useful under some circumstances for the computer to react to 1's and 0's of digital signals and use them in a more direct way to control or regulate the analog world. What we require is an instrument that will take our logic units and convert them into an electrical signal, which is what the digital to analog converter (D/A) performs.

Conceptually, D/A conversion is the inverse of A/D conversion: a digital value is converted to a discrete voltage level, which is smoothed to yield a continuous level of voltage over time. The level of this signal could then be used perhaps after additional analog signal processing—which could consist of amplification, filtering, and signal conditioning—to control some device or affect some action. This is another example of "closing the loop" in which a signal is observed, processed by some algorithm, compared to a standard that yields an output, which then attempts to control the event being observed. These fulfill the requirements of a servomechanism. Computers are finding increasing use as servomechanism devices. There is widespread use of these systems in scientific experimentation and in industrial process control. However, there is still appropriate reluctance to apply servomechanisms as therapeutic devices in humans. A few successful examples include the automatic implantable defibrillator (AID), the glucose controller, and the blood pressure controller. Increasingly powerful hardware and software, coupled with a better understanding of biologic processes, makes it inevitable that more servomechanisms will be applied.

9

Running the Experiment

Up to this point we have covered the necessary steps before beginning the experiment. As the cookbook chapter on preparing hare states, "First catch the hare," so have we laid the foundation for the actual collection of data. Now it's time to examine the process of running the experiment.

WHAT YOU NEED TO KNOW

1. When multiple instruments are assembled to form the instrument chain, the problems and limitations of the whole are more than the sum of the parts.

2. Before data collection begins it is necessary to confirm that the instruments are in proper working order. In addition to routine checks of function, a calibration of electrical and mechanical functions of the instrumentation should be performed on a regular basis.

3. Another type of calibration—signal calibration—is needed each time those data are collected. As a minimum, this calibration will establish the dimensions of the data to be collected and the range and sensitivity (gain) of the system.

4. During the experiment, occasional checking of baseline to correct for drift and instability is desirable, especially in DC-coupled analog instrumentation systems. It also is desirable to recheck signal calibration during or after the experiment.

5. In addition to the rare event of an absolute failure mode, the most severe problem encountered during data collection is the appearance of noise interfering with signal. Noise can be minimized and neutralized, but never banished.

Limitations of the Whole Instrument Chain

There are limitations and problems in the proper operation of the whole chain of instrumentation that may not be apparent in the consideration of individual instruments composing the chain. These include the physical limitations of the space and power requirements, the interference between instruments, and the bandwidth limitations of multiple instruments.

Physical Limitations

It is customary to house instrumentation in one contiguous space so that the investigator can simultaneously calibrate the instruments and monitor their performance during signal measurement. What may start out as an adequate facility to house the experimental preparation and the observer may soon become unwieldy when instruments are added.

Size of Equipment.—One of the positive attributes of modern instruments is their shrinking size. However, adequate space still needs to be allotted for access to and for working with the instruments. Access is especially important when connections between instruments need to be assembled and disassembled, such as cabling, and when the investigator has to make adjustments to the instruments, such as during calibration and at multiple points throughout the experiment.

Power Requirements and Ambient Conditions.—Line-operated instruments may have different power requirements. Although most instrumentation runs on 115 VAC, 60 Hz, some equipment such as treadmills and x-ray generators have higher or multiphase voltage requirements. In addition, there can be differences of operating condition specifications for temperature and humidity between instruments on the one hand and biologic preparations and people on the other. This is especially true for the ambient requirements of some computers that operate in a very limited temperature range. It is usually necessary to house a main computer facility remote from the laboratory while maintaining communication and control by a terminal. Even when equipment does not have stringent environmental specifications, it is quite easy to exceed machine (and human) temperature tolerance when multiple pieces of equipment are assembled in a small space without adequate ventilation. Motors from recorders, cameras, pumps, and treadmills may exceed acoustic tolerance. Clinical facilities and operating rooms may have very stringent fire, safety, and explosion codes that preclude or limit the operation of some instruments.

Ambulatory or Remote Signal Acquisition.—As mentioned in chapter 4, the investigator wants to follow Kelvin's recommendation not to interfere with the signal being measured. Sometimes this will require that the signal source under study be allowed mobility, or not taxed by the limitations of heavy or obstrusive instruments. Additionally, sometimes it is just not feasible for the investigator to be continuously present at the site of the signal source, even though this would ensure continued supervision of the experiment. In such a situation, consider the use of signal telemetry, or small and portable instruments, or instruments that have long-term signal observation and recording properties.

Bandwidth Limitations

It is already obvious that the overall frequency response of an instrumentation chain is limited by the instrument or instruments that limit the high- and low-frequency response of the chain. What is not so obvious is the bandwidth limitation imposed by assembling multiple instruments in series. In such an assembly, the overall frequency response is actually less than that of any single instrument. This effect is shown in the accompanying diagram (Fig 9–1). This occurs because the high-frequency cutoff of each instrument is already reduced 3 dB. The output signal of one instrument becomes the input signal to the next. High-frequency response deteriorates as more instruments are added. When the high-frequency response of one of the instruments is considerably lower than the others (as commonly occurs due to the limited high-frequency response of a transducer or chart recorder) the effect is less but still is considerable.

Turning on the Instruments

It is good practice to develop a checklist or sequence of operations when firing up instruments in preparation for data collection. The con-

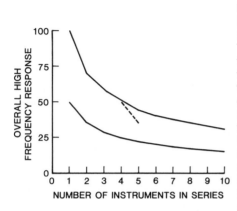

FIG 9–1.
High-frequency response of the instrument chain. When multiple instruments are connected in series, high-frequency response is degraded. The bandwidth limitation that appears at the output of one instrument becomes the input to the next. The solid curve at the top shows the progressive limitation of instrument bandwidth for a series of instruments, each of which has a high-frequency response of 100 Hz (3 dB, or 0.707 of the flat portion of the bandwidth). The dashed line shows the addition of a single instrument with 50 Hz frequency response to four other instruments in series with a 100-Hz response. The solid curve at the bottom is for a series of instruments, each of which has a frequency response of 50 Hz.

cept and practice of this sequence will hold the experimenter in good stead regardless of what new instruments and applications the future holds. The checklist will also contain reminders of the eccentricities of the equipment and the difficulties that are likely to be encountered during the experiment. The steps to be encountered here are the verification of available power, the completeness and the sequence of supplying power to individual instruments, and the duration of warm-up of instruments before use.

Power Source for the Instruments

The first step is to verify that the main power supply is available.

Line Power.—Electricity supplied at the wall outlet—line power—may be controlled by a switch that needs to be turned on. Sometimes, a power indicator light ("idiot" light) or, rarely, a meter will indicate that line power is available.

It is especially convenient to have all instruments of an instrument chain connected to a single power bus controlled by a switch. All power plugs of the individual instruments should be in place before activating the switch in this type of arrangement. Except as noted, electronic instruments may be left in a switched-on condition such that when the power main or bus is activated, all of the instruments will be energized. The exceptions to this are instruments that contain motors or moving parts, and instruments that send or receive start-up (initializing) information from another instrument, and therefore have to be turned on in proper sequence.

Instruments With Motors.—It is advisable to check purposely that each instrument with a motor or moving part is turned off before placing the power plug into an outlet. The windings of motors act as an inductor and produce a back voltage when electrical power is first drawn. If the switch that controls the motor is on, there will be a spark at the outlet when the plug is inserted. A further hazard of instruments containing motors and moving parts is that, if they are turned on unexpectedly, their movement may not be anticipated by personnel, and some untoward mechanical event may occur. The results may vary from amusing to harmful.

Instrument Packages.—Many modern instruments are self-contained packages, in which a single switch activates all components of the package. This is unlikely to be the situation for older equipment, for instruments that have been custom made, and for unique experiments in which multiple rare or exotic instruments have been assembled. Where multiple components are to be switched, they are turned on in stages. First the local power supplies are turned on,* followed by the electronics themselves. Power supplies when first activated are poorly regulated, and surges and uneven voltages are probable. Electronic instruments may be very sensitive to this initial power surge and may be damaged. Even the balkiest power supplies become stable within a few seconds, at which time the electronic components can be turned on.

Sometimes, instruments need to be switched in a particular sequence. This is needed when an instrument provides some start-up information to another instrument at the time it is turned on or, perversely, when it causes some noise or interference. Computer packages consisting of CPU, disk drive, or printer may be especially subject to problems unless switching is in proper sequence.

Warm-up Time.—The time duration necessary for an instrument package to stabilize is a function of the type of instrument in general, and the eccentricity of the instrument in particular. Tube-type instruments, which have all but been abandoned except in very high-power

---

*We recall from chapter 1 that line power is usually 115 VAC, while most instruments use low-power DC. Therefore, a power supply—a device that converts and regulates line power to instrument requirements—will almost always be a component within the cabinet of an instrument.

equipment (x-ray tubes, television monitors), may take a number of seconds or minutes to begin to function or stabilize. They contain "heaters" that regulate electron flow and therefore tube function. In general, the function of all electronic instruments is altered by heat. Since heating is unavoidable, the practice of the instrument manufacturer is to allow heating only within component tolerance, and to achieve a steady state of temperature as soon as possible.

Air vents and fans inside the instrument case and regulation of temperature in the environment assist in both minimizing and stabilizing heating. However, the time to achieve steady-state temperature varies. The proper function of some instrumentation is so sensitive to temperature, for example electronic ovens used in gas analysis, that it is advised to leave them turned on all the time except perhaps when a long period of disuse is anticipated.

Checking Instrument Function Before Use

The scientist should be familiar with the specifications of the instruments being used, as well as their actual performance.

Why Check Instrument Function?

Specified and actual performance of the instrument should coincide, but this is not always so. It may be that instrument performance has deteriorated during use or for lack of maintenance. It may be that instrument performance was never as promised. Equally as likely, published specification of performance may not cover all permutations and combinations of instrument usage, and the scientist may want to confirm performance under the anticipated conditions of the measurements.

Verification of Static Performance

The performance characteristics to be checked during a static calibration of instrument function are the amplitude linearity, range of signal output, and input offset at the available levels of sensitivity.

Input Offset.—Many signals have a reference value: either zero or another absolute value. Instruments may introduce a bias or offset that changes this reference value, or a drift may occur during instrument use. If the reference value is different than expected, or if it changes, then the level of measurement will be incorrect. For example, a vascular pressure measurement is referred to "0" (gauge or ambient) pressure. If an instrument introduces a bias or a baseline drift of the reference pressure, then the level of the measurement of pressure will be wrong (Fig 9–2).

Input offset is checked in one or two steps. First a zero electrical signal is applied at the most proximal instrument in the chain that accepts an electrical input. For example, the input to the amplifier is turned off or shorted while the level of the output is observed. If required, the output level is adjusted to zero or reference level by the offset suppression adjustment of the amplifier. Next, if possible and appropriate, the signal detector is added to the instrument chain. A signal that is intended to mimic or model biologic zero or reference is applied to the detector while the output level of the instrument chain

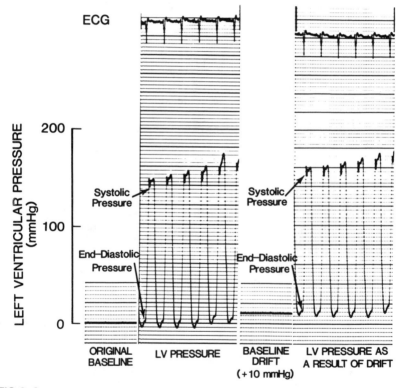

FIG 9–2.
Effect of amplifier drift. The strain gauge used for measurement of left ventricular pressure is referenced to a zero pressure level *(left panels)*. During the course of the measurements, there was a drift so that the reference pressure increased by 10 mm Hg. This artifactually appeared to increase the measured pressure *(right panels)*. The correct procedure is to reestablish the reference zero pressure.

is observed. If required, the output level is adjusted to zero or reference by an additional offset suppression adjustment. Various names are applied to this adjustment. On a strain gauge amplifier it is called the balance knob. If a zero or reference cannot be obtained, the instrument is probably broken. Sometimes, the reference value is not zero or cannot be adjusted to zero. In that case, one makes a note of the level of the reference and corrects the level of the measurement to the reference level after acquiring the data.

Amplitude Linearity.—It is expected that the level of the signal will vary during the observation period, and that this signal level will be amplified—usually greatly increased—by the instrumentation. Therefore, it is important to know the constancy of the sensitivity of the system over the expected range of the signal. This is called amplitude linearity. In graphical terms, we are observing the constancy of the slope of the sensitivity of the system. In chapter 3, we discussed amplitude linearity as one of the sources of nonrandom error during measurement. If there is deviation from amplitude linearity, then different levels of the signal will be amplified at different gains, and there will be distortion of the levels of the signal.

Amplitude linearity is checked by applying and maintaining a static input signal level at a specified sensitivity while observing the output of the instrument. Observation at one extreme of the range is made (either the high or low end), then the level of the signal is serially adjusted to another level throughout the range. If hysteresis is suspected (chapter 3), then a series of observations is made first starting from one end of the range and then the other. The input signal is applied for a long enough period of time to allow the ouput to come to a steady state. By sweeping the signal level over the range, and observing variation of the output from the expected, one is measuring the amplitude linearity of the instrument at a particular sensitivity. By sweeping signal level from one end of the range to the other and back again and observing variation of the output from the expected, one is measuring hysteresis.

During a series of measurements, more than one level of sensitivity may be used. At the time of analysis, the signal measured at the different sensitivities will be compared. Therefore it is important to know how the different nominal levels of gain (the named values that appear on the sensitivity or gain control of the instrument) affect the level of the signal. It is also common that the scientist will find that but a single level of sensitivity is all that is intended to be used during a series of observations. Even so, it is worthwhile to see what happens during an additional static calibration that is applied to other levels of sensitivity (usually a factor of two) higher and lower than the expected level of sensitivity.

The relationship between different levels of sensitivity in the same instrument is performed by the application of a test signal at midrange level of a particular sensitivity. Sensitivity adjustments are made higher and lower than the starting sensitivity. If the next adjustment of sensitivity is twofold that of the present level, the output should be double the original output. If the next adjustment of sensitivity is half that of the present level, the output should be half of the original output. This check is important because the investigator will want to maximize use of the scale resolution by altering sensitivity applied to the signal. If the investigator changes sensitivity during signal measurement, and the output does not change as the exact ratio of the nominal (expected) values of the sensitivity, an error may occur unless additional calibrations are performed.

Range and Scale.—At the same time that a calibration of amplitude linearity and sensitivity is performed, it is customary to check that the range and scale of operation will be sufficient for that intended. Sometimes, the signal level will not optimally use the range of the instrument. Small signals will be near the lower limit of the range. When coupled with a limited resolution of the scale, it may not be feasible to measure different levels of the signal. Occasionally, the signal will be too large, and a clipped output will make it impossible to measure different levels of the signal. This check is performed by applying a high and low test signal level and observing where the output falls with respect to the range limit.

Verification of Dynamic Performance
Just as it is desirable to check static performance, it is also desirable to check dynamic performance, or bandwidth.

Calibration of Bandwidth.—A full test of dynamic range (as opposed to calibration of high and low cutoff frequencies or natural frequency) requires carefully calibrated and appropriate test instruments. The test instruments produce a bandwidth of sine waves that are applied as inputs to the instrument chain. A function generator is an appropriate test instrument. Its sine wave output can be applied as an electrical test signal to the input of an amplifier or a recorder—that is, instruments that can accept an electrical input. For example, I used sine waves generated by a function generator to calibrate the frequency response of the chart recorders discussed in chapter 7 (see Fig 7–1).

The test equipment and the procedure for this are simple and straight-forward.

Dynamic calibration gets stickier when one attempts to measure the bandwidth of a transducer: you have to duplicate the energy form of the signal input to the transducer. Very few investigators have access to a sinusoidal pressure generator for a test of pressure transducer bandwidth, or a sinusoidal flow generator for a test of a flow transducer bandwidth. If you do have the access to test instruments and the technical expertise to apply them, I recommend that you perform this determination of bandwidth a single time when the instruments are first assembled. The results can be a real eye opener.

As an example, I used a hydraulic function generator to calibrate a transducer. A series of calibrations was performed on a fluid-filled strain gauge pressure transducer alone, with the pressure transducer attached to two different intravascular catheters, and with small air bubbles introduced into the assembly (Fig 9–3). Note that, in general, the high-frequency response of the transducer is degraded by the addition of a catheter or an air bubble. However, the exception is that a short-bore catheter actually improved the frequency response of the transducer alone. The actual types of frequency response I observed are close to that predicted from theoretical models of the behavior of second-order systems (see chapter 3, Fig 3–2). This includes resonance and attenuation of the system. However, the exact behavior of a particular system required calibration of the system.

Obviously, this calibration includes most of the contingencies to be found in biologic measurement, and is the calibration of choice. Why is this rigorous calibration not employed routinely, and only dwelt on in textbooks and review articles? Two reasons: the dynamic pressure calibration system is difficult and moderately expensive to build, apply, and maintain; and most experimenters are either naive or believe that they are knowledgeable about the bandwidth of their instruments. They may also infer that the bandwidth of the signal under investigation is well within the frequency response of the instruments used to measure that signal. That may or may not be true. Compromise is possible between these two positions. It is most appropriate when assembling an instrumentation chain, or changing any of its components, to review bandwidth specifications and to consider a calibration of frequency response. Once performed, it is acceptable to rely on static calibration and to be confident that the stability of the dynamic response has not changed.

To see how this calibration of frequency response translates into the distortion of a signal, I recorded a pulmonary artery pressure. First, the signal was recorded with the pressure transducer and flotation

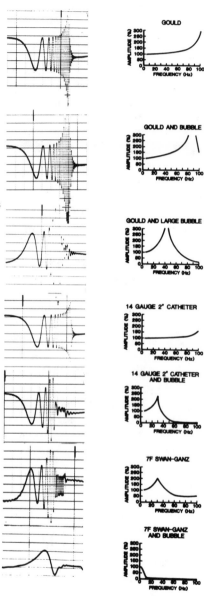

FIG 9–3.
Frequency response of a fluid-filled pressure transducer. A dynamic pressure generator was used to calibrate the frequency response of (from top to bottom) a pressure transducer; the transducer with a small air bubble introduced into its fluid column; the transducer with a larger air bubble; the transducer with a short and stiff catheter (14-gauge Teflon catheter, 2 in long); the transducer with the catheter and an air bubble; the transducer and a balloon flotation catheter; the transducer with the catheter and an air bubble. Notice that the frequency response of the system deteriorated with the air bubbles and the balloon flotation catheter, but actually improved with the short catheter. The types of changes of frequency response, as anticipated from chapter 2, were either resonance, attenuation, or both.

catheter shown in the next-to-the-bottom panel of Figure 9–3. Then, I introduced a small air bubble to simulate the alterations of frequency response shown in the bottom panel of Figure 9–3. The results are shown in the accompanying figure (Fig 9–4). Note that the system without the bubble has an adequate frequency response to record higher frequencies in the signal, such as the dicrotic notch and "a" wave. When a bubble is introduced, the amplitude of the high frequencies is dampened or attenuated, congruent with our calibration data. This example illustrates that the investigator usually treads on a fine line when it comes to frequency response. You must heed not only the specifications of the instrument as it comes from the box, but also the alterations that may occur in actual use.

Signal Calibration

Calibration of the signal serves the important function of providing the proper biologic dimensions to the observations and reducing the level of nonrandom error.

PRESSURE TRANSDUCER AND 7F RIGHT HEART CATHETER

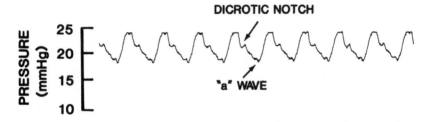

PRESSURE TRANSDUCER, 7F RIGHT HEART CATHETER AND SMALL AIR BUBBLE

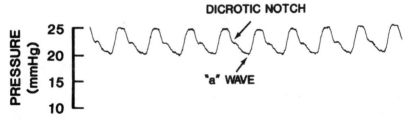

FIG 9–4.
Frequency response of a catheter-manometer system during pressure measurement. The system of the next-to-the-bottom panel of Figure 9–3 was used to measure pulmonary artery pressure *(top panel)*. It is known that the dicrotic notch and the "a" wave of this signal have high frequencies. Then, a small air bubble was introduced into the system. There is a degraded high-frequency response of the system as predicted from Figure 9–3, with a reduction of the amplitude of the dicrotic notch and "a" wave.

Providing Dimensions to the Data

The instrumentation discussed in this book accepts as an input a variety of biologic signals—bioelectricity, pressure, flow, motion, photon emission, or the signal from another instrument—and provides an electrical output. There are rare exceptions to this, but the point is that the output of the instrument chain is *usually not* in biologic dimensions such as mm Hg, L/min, or ml of end-diastolic volume. In that case, the scientist takes some pains to simulate some input signal that will mimic or be an analogy of the biologic signal, in order to relate the signal that comes out of the instrumentation chain to the one that went into it. These calibration signals take two forms: signals with the same dimensions of the biologic signal to be measured, and signals of electrical equivalence to the output stage of some instrument early in the instrumentation chain (usually a transducer).

Calibration Signals With Dimensions of Biologic Signals.—These are the preferred form of calibration signal because they encompass the largest portion of the instrument chain, and because they most closely simulate the biologic signal. The goal is to apply the signal at the very front end of the instrumentation chain, that is, where the instrumentation chain interfaces with the signal source. A signal is applied, and the output of the system is observed. The output could be a deflection of a pen on a recorder, or a change in the number of a display device, or a voltage deflection that will be recorded on a magnetic tape or entered on a computer. The ratio of output to input is called the overall gain or the sensitivity of the system.

For example, we want to measure arterial blood pressure and have assembled a transducer, strain gauge amplifier, instrumentation amplifier and filter, and a pen writing recorder. By use of a mercury manometer, we apply a known pressure at the input port of the pressure transducer—say 100 mm Hg—and observe a pen deflection on the strip chart recorder of perhaps 10 cm. We say that the overall gain or sensitivity of the system is 10 cm of deflection per 100 mm Hg (signal output/signal input). Note that in this type of calibration, gain has dimensions (cm/mm Hg), although this is not always the case—for instance, if the output and input signals have the same dimension. The level of an unknown pressure is determined by the distance of pen deflection away from baseline or zero, divided by the overall system gain. If the deflection in this example were 7 cm away from baseline, then the pressure would be 70 mm Hg (7 cm/[10 cm/100 mm Hg]).

It is also worthwhile to make two additional points. First, our calibration signal, although entered near the front of the instrumentation chain, was not truly at the very front. That is, in order to measure pressure with a fluid-filled strain gauge manometer, it is necessary to connect the pressure source (blood vessel in this case) to the manometer with a tube or catheter. It is frequently not convenient to attach the calibration source to the transducer through the catheter. It is customary for the experimenter to "forgive" this assumption and to assume that the intervening device would not cause a deviation in the calibration. This raises the second point: most calibrations are static, whereas most biologic signals are dynamic. Given our previous discussions on frequency response, including alterations of amplitude and phase, it is possible that static calibration will not adequately simulate biologic reality.

Calibration Signals of Electrical Equivalence.—Sometimes, a physical analogy of the signal is forgone in favor of an electrical analogy. This type of calibration signal is used when it is very difficult to apply a physical signal, or when the biologic signal is electrical in the first place, or when the instrument sensitivity has been established with certainty as constant.

Sometimes, it is very difficult to get to the front of the instrumentation chain and provide a physical calibration signal. Consider thermodilution cardiac output instrumentation. The physical analogy for calibration might be a water bath of known temperature that could be applied to the thermistor, and measured as a deflection on a pen writing recorder. This type of calibration was actually performed in the not-too-distant past. However, it is impractical and untidy to provide such a calibration. Instead, an equivalent electrical signal, equal to that of a temperature (change) of the thermistor, is provided at an early stage in the instrumentation chain, but after the thermistor, in order to establish calibration. This type of calibration is accurate only if the sensitivity (electrical output/temperature input) of the instrumentation in front of this calibration signal is known with certainty and is stable. Thermistors are extremely reliable transducers that can be adjusted at the time of manufacture to have a known and stable calibration. Under these circumstances, a simulation by an electrical analogy has proven feasible. Contrariwise, most instrumentation engineers do not feel as secure about calibrating thermocouples by a signal of electrical equivalence, unless great pains are taken to stabilize the thermocouple reference junction. This is one reason why thermistors are more frequently used in biologic work.

Solid-state manometers mounted on a catheter tip are another example of an instrument where it is possible and desirable to use an electrical calibration signal as a substitute for a biologic signal. Although it is possible to calibrate the catheter-tipped manometer with a pressure while it is outside the body, this is not possible once it is passed into its position of measurement. Two alternatives have been used. In one case, a fluid-filled catheter (connected to an external manometer) is passed to the same measuring site as the catheter-tipped manometer. The pressure from the fluid-filled catheter (especially the low-frequency diastolic pressure) is used to calibrate the catheter-tipped manometer. Admittedly, this sounds a little crazy. The other alternative is to rely on the original ex vivo calibration. Some solid-state manometers have a very stable sensitivity, so that there is a known change of electrical output for a given change of pressure signal input. Contrariwise, drift and temperature stability have been problematic with these manometers.

Reducing Noise and Interference During Measurement

In its broadest definition, error is any signal that is recorded other than the signal of interest. Here, we are addressing a specific type of error called *random error*. In instrumentation parlance, this is called *noise* or *interference*. The worst possible time to become aware of noise is during the conduct of the experiment. It is preferable and possible to be aware of noise and to reduce noise before the actual collection of data.

Noise Theory

The signal-to-noise ratio (N) is a useful engineering term that expresses the level of noise in a system in reference to the level of signal. In the case of electronic instruments, noise is expressed as a voltage equivalent. Because both noise and signal may have positive or negative levels that oscillate around zero over time, the simple average of either could be misleading and may even result in a value of zero. This would result in a quotient for N of either zero or infinity. We have encountered this before as a similar problem in the calculation of "effective" AC electrical values (see chapter 1). Therefore, both signal and noise levels are squared. If the ratio of the values squared is calculated (mean square), then N is said to have been determined on a power basis. If the square root of this squared value is calculated (root mean square), then N is said to have been determined on an amplitude basis. Sometimes, it does not make sense to calculate the square of the signal, and the quotient of N will have a numerator that expresses the energy of the signal while the denominator will be the mean square energy noise.

The higher the ratio the better, although no minimum acceptable value for N can be given; that depends upon the experimental conditions and the techniques used for data analysis. For example, multiple methods of analysis may allow relatively low values of N to realize acceptable results. Also, if signal averaging techniques can be applied, then any value of N may be acceptable. The application of signal averaging is limited only by the duration and reliability of the experimental preparation.

Noise can originate from many sources (Table 9–1). For the purpose of classification, we partition noise by site of production into two categories: internal noise and external noise.

Internal Noise

Internal noise is that noise generated within the source of the biologic signal or within the instrumentation chain.

Instrument Noise.—There are a number of sources of noise produced within instruments, including noise from amplifiers and signal detectors. Amplifiers are associated with thermal (Johnson) noise, shot and partition noise, current noise, and bursts. Some of these are proportional to the bandwidth of the instruments and some are independent of the bandwidth. This is an example of where purposely limiting instrument bandwidth to that required by the biologic signal is beneficial.

Amplifier noise is usually less than electrode noise (battery-like po-

TABLE 9–1.

Sources of Noise

TYPE	EXAMPLES	COMMENTS
Internal noise		
Instrument	Amplifier, electrode	Some proportional to bandwidth
Biologic	Heart, skeletal muscle	Localize site of recording
External noise		
Electrical	Electrostatic, electromagnetic, direct	Remove sources, ground instruments and subjects, provide shielding
Mechanical	Vibration	Remove sources or move site of experiment; shock mount instruments

tentials, spikes and drift). Selection of low-noise electrodes, and waiting a few minutes after the application of electrodes for stabilization of battery discharge, can greatly reduce electrode noise.

Biologic Noise.—Biologic systems carry on many different functions at the same time, accompanied by changing electrical potentials, vibration and temperature changes. Because an experimenter wishes to record a discrete signal, these other signals are then considered noise.

Mechanical interference can transfer energy to a mechanical or electrical transducer. For example, the catheter whip seen in a fluid-filled catheter can induce a substantial pressure artifact. Also, the motion of walking or cycling can induce a large electrical interference signal in electrodes used for bioelectric events.

Electrical interference from biologic sources can be of either large or small amplitude. Large amplitude interference is seen when one bioelectric signal grossly contaminates the bioelectric source of interest, such as when the ECG or EMG is seen on the EEG signal. Small amplitude interference is caused by multiple small alterations of bioelectric phenomena, such as alterations in resting membrane potential, which may produce changes in recorded bioelectric phenomena.

External Noise

Outside noise or interference is the main source of noise during signal acquisition. This noise enters the recording system apart from or in combination with the signal. The two types are electrical and mechanical.

Electrical Interference.—There are three ways in which electrical interference is coupled to an amplifier—electrostatic (capacitive coupled), electromagnetic (inductively coupled), and direct (resistively coupled). We have previously described all three as capable of causing microshock hazards (see chapter 1). Here, we will discuss them in terms of noise. The same procedures can be used to eliminate these sources as shock and noise potentials.

In electrostatic coupling (capacitive coupling), a source of high potential gains access to the input terminals of the amplifier. The most ubiquitous and frequently the largest amplitude source occurs from 60 Hz electrical power lines. We are literally surrounded by these sources, such as high-voltage cables, fluorescent lamps, and transformers. All instrument cases and conductors (including biologic tissues and humans) act as antennas. This source of amplifier input voltage and electrical hazard is completely eliminated when a properly grounded shield is placed between the source of potential and the input terminals of the amplifier. The most effective form of shielding, but one that is unwieldy and many times impractical, is a cage placed around the biologic preparation and the instrumentation and attached to ground—a Faraday cage. If the signal is a bioelectric potential, a large amount of electrostatic coupling can be eliminated by proper selection and preparation of the site of the ground electrode. This connection may be more feasible than any source of shielding.

Electromagnetic interference also includes radio frequency interference. This type of interference is inductively coupled to the input stage of the amplifier. Electromagnetic sources include AC power lines, and the current changes produced by switching on and off motors, solenoids, transformers, and thermostats. Radio frequency sources include radio, television, and short-wave signals as well as motors and other spark-generating equipment. Computers have become the latest and one of the most ubiquitous sources of radio frequency interference. A simple but effective method to reduce magnetic interference is to twist the input wires of the amplifier together. Radio frequency interference is also greatly lessened by electrostatic shielding of the instrument case and the cable, because the shield destroys the original phase relation of the radio frequency. Massive electromagnetic screening is largely impractical. If a further step is necessary to decrease interference, these sources should be removed as far as possible from the amplifier.

Resistive interference occurs when a potential is generated through a poorly devised grounding system resulting in a ground loop. This occurs when two or more grounds are brought to earth through different paths. This is possible where, for example, the ground connected to the electrical power conduit has been connected to a cold water pipe that enters the earth, while a separate ground connection such as a spike driven into the earth has been created. If both grounds are used for two different pieces of equipment or for a device and the indifferent lead of the biologic tissue, then the large cross-sectional area contained between the ground loop causes heavy electromagnetic pickup. The current flowing through even a small resistance will induce a voltage and will be amplified the same way as the real input signal. This is eliminated by removing the ground loop and bringing all ground lines from equipment and biologic tissue to a single ground.

Mechanical Interference.—Electronic devices are largely immune from small amounts of mechanical energy, and from the induced electrical voltage of mechanical vibration. Where a vibrating source contacts equipment, the application of protection through damping with materials that lead to a much higher natural frequency than that encountered will aid in this problem. The only other alternative is to move the experimental site far from the source of vibration.

Preparing for Noise and Interference

Awareness of Environment.—It is helpful for the experimenter to be aware of the noise environment in which the data are to be collected. The presence of other equipment and personnel, and the likely times and manner in which other equipment is used, may allow you to identify noise problems. Large pieces of equipment that could generate interference—whether electrical or mechanical—are worth noting. For example, any large transformer or power-generating equipment is likely to cause interference. New sources at the top of the current list are magnetic resonance imaging instruments, which generate radio frequency and magnetic fields, and computers and digital devices, which generate radio frequency interference. Large rotating mechanical equipment, such turbines and generators, can also be troublesome.

Equipment that is connected on the same power line, whether from your laboratory or someone else's, can be a problem. This is especially true for equipment that contains motors or generates radio frequency signals and that periodically switches on and off such as refrigerators, centrifuges, x-ray equipment, and elevators.

Equipment Dry Run.—The instrument chain should be assembled in the place and position in which it is to be used. Other environmental sources of interference, such as fluorescent lighting and the personnel and equipment of other laboratories, should be simulating their normal activities. It is advisable to first remove any (mechanical) display writing recorder from the instrumentation chain, and replace it with a non-mechanical device capable of wide bandwidth, such as an oscilloscope. This will not only save paper, galvanometers, and pens, but will also permit maximum observation of noise. Subsequently, if noise levels are low, the output of the instrument chain should be directed toward the normal display device, such as a pen writing recorder.

After the equipment is switched on and allowed to warm up (see above) the inputs of the amplifiers should be shorted, and the output observed on the display devices. The user should perform this at least twice. First, the settings of the equipment should be at the widest bandwidth, that is, filter, amplifier, and recorder settings should be left at the widest frequency response, even if these are not the intended settings for the experiment. After initial observations are made at the amplifier gain (sensitivity) settings that are anticipated during the experiment, the gain settings should be increased and noise observed. From this, the user will have the opportunity to observe the maximum type and sources of all regularly occurring noise events. Although some of these events may have a small amplitude, it could be that these are minimal events at the time of observation with the possibility of wider fluctuations at other times. The observations should be repeated a second time with the bandwidth of the equipment adjusted to those settings anticipated during the experiment. This will provide a more realistic appraisal of the amount of noise that is likely to be present during the experiment.

10

Maintenance and Repair

A voice said, Look me in the stars
And tell me truly, men of earth
If all the soul-and-body scars
Were not too much to pay for birth.
                    *Robert Frost**

One of the most frustrating and unrewarding parts of dealing with an instrument is its inevitable failure, and the ensuing process of repair. Modern instrumentation is remarkably failure free, although the novice scientist may find himself the beneficiary of older, more imperfect equipment. In anticipation of future problems, it would do you well to be prepared ahead of time. In some circumstances, the problems with instrument function can be averted by preventive maintenance. In other circumstances, the problems are minor and may be readily corrected. However, a catastrophic failure of instrument function, despite the best of efforts to prevent it, may provide a challenge to your patience and pocketbook.

WHAT YOU NEED TO KNOW

1. Assemble vital manuals and spare parts so that they are readily accessible.

2. Maintain equipment and, for some instruments, consider buying preventive maintenance contracts and service contracts.

3. Troubleshoot the problem within your capacity in order to define, delimit, and possibly self-repair the instrument.

Assemble Helpful Material

You need to make some preparations in anticipation of instrument usage, let alone maintenance and repair. Materials on hand should include manuals, supplies, and simple spare parts. Additionally, some consideration needs to be given to who, how, and where service will be performed on instruments in need of maintenance and service.

Where does one get information to help you prepare for the usage, maintenance, and repair of an instrument? In addition to the manufacturer, there is major assistance available from sales representatives or distributors, as well as independent service organizations. During the course of instrument purchase and usage, you may have more contact with the sales representative or distributor than the manufacturer. That person or company may provide you with a high degree of personalized service and competent advice, and their name, address, and telephone number should be kept on file.

Manuals

There are two types of manuals that the instrument manufacturer publishes that contain information a user will require. They are the *operations* manual and the *repair* manual. These manuals should be complete and comprehensible for their intended purpose. Unfortunately, this may not be the case. Many third parties have published books and made their fortunes based on explaining how something works and how to use it—witness this book.

Operations Manual.—The operations manual always is supplied with the instrument, and provides instructions on the operating principles of the equipment and details of setup, calibration, and safe operation. It also includes the name, address and telephone number of the manufacturer, and, if others are authorized to provide a service for the instrument, the names and addresses of distributors, parts suppliers and repair centers.

Repair and Maintenance Manual.—The repair and maintenance manual contains a schematic (circuit diagram) of the electrical and electronic design, a parts list, and sometimes specific technical information on maintenance and repair operations. It may be included as part of the operations manual, or it may be separate. In addition to an actual manual, the schematic itself may be printed on a sheet of paper and pasted somewhere within the case of the instrument. Sometimes the manual has to be specifically ordered and paid for apart from instrument purchase, particularly if a second copy is needed. To show you how important this is, the manual usually has a "part #" designation just like the op amps, motors, and gizmos of the instrument!

The first question any technician will ask when confronted with a repair is, "Where's the schematics?"—that is, where is the electronic circuit diagram, parts list, and critical test and validation points of the electrical circuit. If you don't have this manual, you're not going to get much enthusiasm from service people unless they are intimately familiar with the instrument or have access to the repair manual themselves.

Supplies and Parts

Supplies.—Supplies are considered to be parts that will be consumed during normal instrument operation. Of course, for a writing recorder, one is going to keep a supply of chart paper on hand; if it's an ink-writing recorder one will also have a supply of ink. Be wary of hoarding spare supplies that have a limited lifespan such as photographic paper, batteries, and chemicals, since they may expire and be useless before they are needed.

Parts, Tools, and Test Equipment.—At a minimum, one should have some tools and simple test equipment in order to make simple adjustments and to perform preliminary troubleshooting (described below). The tools you'll need include screwdrivers (slotted, Phillips, and Torx), small wrenches (English and metric), a soldering iron, test leads (temporary connectors and cables), and a VOM (volt-ohm-ammeter). If you can buy or inherit an oscilloscope, it will prove very valuable. If you employ a technical person who is expert in doing advanced repairs, you'll have to up the ante of the amount of equipment kept on hand.

It also is advisable to keep some parts that are used for repair on hand. Usually a little insight is all that is needed to see what should be kept on hand and what can be ordered at the time of failure. Any inexpensive mechanical part should be stocked; pens, fuses, cables, and batteries are examples. Decisions about more expensive and less-frequently broken parts require individual judgment. Often in the course of a repair, a used but operable part will be salvaged. Find some place to save it to use for emergency repairs. Contrariwise, don't save any part that's not operational. It will find its way back into the instrument and cause endless confusion.

Storing Manuals, Supplies, and Parts

Someone is going to have to be responsible for the safekeeping of these manuals, supplies, tools, test equipment and spare parts. It is highly desirable to keep some supplies and parts (paper, ink, pens and fuses) and the operations manual at the location of the instrument itself. Since it is used much less frequently, and bound to be misplaced, it is recommended to keep the repair manual in a known library of technical information. If you have a reliable instrumentation repair department, leave the manual with them.

Some items which are irregularly used, and whose shelf life is prolonged by refrigeration (some chemicals, photographic paper and batteries), may be kept remote from their site of use. Some spare parts need to be kept with the people who are qualified to actually use them during repair. Keep a list of where everything is, and its expiration date.

Repair and Maintenance

The instrument user is confronted by a 2×2 contingency table when it comes to repair and maintenance (Table 10–1): there are two choices of who is going to do the work (in-house or out-of-house) and two choices of when the repair work will be done (preventive maintenance or as needed).

Who Will Do the Work?

Unless you have the communication skills and luck of a Tom Sawyer, you're going to have to plan ahead to identify who will repair and maintain your equipment.

In-house Repair.—Usually the most effective and efficient way of getting something done is to do it yourself, or to have someone you trust do it. However, most people responsible for data collection just don't have the time and skill to maintain and repair their instruments.

TABLE 10–1.
Contingency Table for Repair and Maintenance

	SOURCE OF REPAIR	
	IN-HOUSE	CONTRACTOR
Advantages	Easy to contact	Special experience
	Less expensive	Efficient repair
	Possible to verify progress	Possible loan instrument
Disadvantages	Poorly responsive	Offsite repair
	Lack of special parts	Expensive
	TYPE OF REPAIR	
	PREVENTIVE MAINTENANCE	REPAIR WHEN BROKEN
Advantages	Limit complete breakdowns	Avoid unnecessary down time
	Improved operation	Less expensive
	Early response to breakdowns and possible equipment loan	Early response to breakdowns
Disadvantages	May create problems	Unexpected disruption of operation
	High fixed cost	Unpredictable cost

At a minimum, some responsibility will have to devolve onto the investigator; otherwise, every time a roll of paper needs to be changed the measurements will have to stop—a most unsatisfactory arrangement.

The most satisfactory, but expensive, alternative is to have an instrumentation specialist directly responsible for your needs. Usually this person services the instruments of a few investigators or a department. If highly skilled, the specialist not only repairs and maintains instruments, but also designs and builds custom instrumentation. It has become very difficult to obtain intramural or extramural funding for this type of specialist.

Under some circumstances, it is highly satisfactory to have maintenance and repair performed by an organization within your institution. Most larger institutions have an instrument repair and model shop, whose purpose it is to maintain and repair equipment and to fabricate custom instrumentation. It pays to be on good terms with this crew, and to recognize the beleaguered position in which this department usually finds itself: they are usually understaffed, and they are subject to the abuse that everyone needs their equipment fixed *now*. Usually, institutions set up some priorities on instrument repair; for instance, the highest priority is given to repair of instruments used in patient-care areas, while the lowest priority is assigned to the fabrication of custom instruments (unless you can get the assigned instrumentation technician interested in your project). A frank discussion with this department as to matching your needs with their capabilities and time alllocation will allow you to prepare an appropriate plan of who will care for your instruments.

Out-of-house Repairs.—Sometimes there is good reason to go outside your institution to have your instrument maintained or repaired.

One source of out-of-house repairs is the manufacturer or manufacturer's authorized service. You may consider this contingency if the time and capabilities of in-house people are going to be unsuitable or inconstant. Some instruments may demand special attention for maintenance and repair, because they contain proprietary parts or unusual service needs. This translates into a requirement for factory-authorized service by a small number of specialists with access to special parts and test equipment. When you are considering buying or borrowing such an instrument (see chapter 11), be wary of this possibility since it may require a commitment that you are unwilling or unhappy about making. However, the trade-off for this limitation of repair options may include a loan of a substitute piece of equipment by the authorized repair center. Because these services are profit making, and because customer satisfaction may be linked to future patronage and sales, repair by the manufacturer or authorized service center may be prompt, efficient, and courteous.

It may also be wise to consider independent, local repair centers. Usually, these were started as one-man shops by a technician who was moonlighting from his regular employment, working in his garage at night and on weekends, and accessed by customers through irregular channels. Although such informal and less expensive arrangements still exist, many of these operations have become fully staffed, storefront operations and are accessed by customers through regular channels. The profit motive and promise of your return for service may make them very reliable.

When Should Repairs Be Performed?

The user has two choices in this regard: preventive maintenance or as needed.

Preventive Maintenance.—The concept of preventive maintenance is that equipment will break or foul in a relatively known way in a relatively defined time. From this, one should be able to predict when and where in an instrument to intervene to replace, repair, or clean the instrument so as to prevent its abrupt and untimely failure during usage.

There is some truth to this notion under a few circumstances. The single most important consideration is safety maintenance. I need to restate bluntly what we indicated in chapter 1: that electrical safety and other aspects of instrument safety are a house of cards ready to collapse on our patients and ourselves unless we take the greatest care. Institutions may be required by governmental codes, regulating authorities, and internal policy to have a program of safety maintenance and to keep detailed records of this program.

In addition to safety maintenance, instruments that have mechanical parts, that operate in a dirty environment, or that generate materials that tend to foul their operation should be considered for preventive maintenance. Also, instruments that have been observed by the user or the manufacturer to fail in a known way and in a known time are also candidates for preventive maintenance. Some insight into this may be gained by reading the operations and repair manual. If a long list of suggested maintenance tasks is required, it may be prudent to consider preventive maintenance.

Preventive maintenance can be performed either in house or out of house. To save money, you may consider performing this on your own or with the support of your colleagues. The in-house instrumentation shop may be able to help; however, few in-house instrumentation shops can afford the time for preventive maintenance of all the instruments in an institution. In that situation, it may be wise to consider preventive maintenance by the manufacturer, an authorized service dealer, or by an independent repair agency. However, the success of such a program depends on the familiarity of the service personnel with the type of instrument, its eccentricities and failure modes, and its suggested maintenance program.

Another reason to consider preventive maintenance is because it may be linked in some way to instrument repair. For example, some service contracts provide preventive maintenance in the anticipation that this will lessen the number and types of repair. This will reduce contractor costs and increase customer satisfaction. Some users believe it is easier to get rapid repair service out of a dealer or representative who is supplying preventive maintenance, because the contractor feels responsible for the operation of the instrument. However, it is also likely that a contractor will respond to the sudden appearance of a new cash customer, and defer service on the instrument of an existing customer who has a paid-up contract.

Repair When Broken.—There are some limitations to the concept of preventive maintenance. As a medical student, I worked with an intern who, when he finished with a patient would say to them, "You're good for another six months or 6,000 miles, whichever comes first." Ah, if the ills of people or instruments only were so simple. The failure or fouling of an instrument may not be predictable or preventable. Also, careless maintenance runs the risk of causing new problems during the course of the maintenance. What is suggested here is that it may be suitable to wait for an instrument failure (other than safety failure) before undertaking repair. It is advised that some preparations be made ahead of time for rapidly effecting repair when it is needed.

Summary.—In the foregoing discussion I have presented two contrary viewpoints on preventive maintenance and repair. The most that can be suggested is that each instrument is different.

Getting Service
Paying for Instrument Repair.—Someone has to pay for these repairs, and unless your grant or your Dean has made some provision, you'll have to face the reality of these costs. Service contracts bear especially close scrutiny.

Service Contracts.—Contracts for maintenance and repair are available from authorized and independent service dealers. As with all contracts, read the fine print. The fine print should include a description of what type of work is to be performed, where the work is to be performed, how quickly it will be performed, and whether a loan of equipment is available while yours is "down."

Contracts may be only for repair service, which means you'll see the service representative only if you make a call and report that something has gone wrong. Preventive maintenance plus repair specifies that the service representative will deliver maintenance based on some schedule—perhaps elapsed time or hours of usage—plus repair when called.

Service may be performed on site, which means that repair will occur where the equipment is; or, by depot, which means that you must deliver the instrument to the repair center. Obviously, a large or very fragile instrument must be serviced on site. However, it has become popular for small instruments, such as microcomputers, to require delivery to the contractor's service center. If the contract calls for depot, and the service center is not nearby, shipping the instrument will cause a delay of repair and a freight and insurance cost.

A deadline should be included in a contract and indicates the outside limit of time the contractor has before the repair must be completed. Without such a clause, you could wait weeks or months before repair is completed. Such a clause is worthless unless it includes a provision for a financial penalty to the contractor—something that they really wouldn't want to happen to them.

Loaners and backups mean that while your instrument is under repair, or should a repair deadline be missed, the contractor will provide a working instrument under loan. There may be a fee for this, but at least you'll keep going. It's important that the loaned instrument reproduce the specifications of the instrument under repair. This may not be possible for certain custom or rare species of instruments.

Do-It-Yourself Instrument Maintenance and Repair

There are some maintenance and repair items which the user can perform simply and expeditiously. They may save you the cost of maintenance and repair, and the wasted time obligated by a broken instrument.

Instrument Maintenance

Keep Instruments Clean.—Most equipment has very narrow tolerances of operating conditions. Any foreign or residual material from the environment or from the byproducts of usage may impair performance. Unlike the dishes, which can be left in the kitchen sink until the day after the party, it is prudent to clean up immediately after using an instrument.

It should be absolutely forbidden to bring food or drink into the area of equipment—no matter what the duration of the measurements! And the horror of the adverse health and performance effects of second-hand cigarette smoke on personnel, the fouling of instruments by cigarette ashes, and the danger of fire from smoking cannot be overemphasized.

Don't Block Ventilation.—Most equipment produces heat in operation, and most components, especially electrical ones, only have a limited tolerance for heating before failure occurs. Manufacturers usually provide vents on cabinets to allow convective transfer of heat to the environment. These vents are usually on the top and sides of the case, and can be covered inadvertently by papers, books, or other instruments.

Equipment that produces a higher thermal load—more heat—will use an internal cooling fan. Again, special care must be taken to avoid blocking the intake and output ports of the fan. In rare circumstances, especially those involving engines, a coolant other than air is used. The maintenance and care of these coolant systems introduces another level of complexity into equipment maintenance and repair.

Run the Instruments Every Day.—Under rare circumstances, some equipment should be used daily, even when measurements are not being made. This is especially true for pen writing recorders, which have a tendency to clog unless used daily, or for other devices that contain finicky mechanical parts. Some instrument users also subscribe to the concept that equipment failures tend to be random, and it would be best to detect a fault on a day off rather than the day of the actual experiment.

Leave Instruments on Continuously.—Some equipment is best left on continuously. In some instruments, thermal stability is extremely important for function, and this is only achieved after a number of hours of operation.

Anticipate Instrument Failure.—The best circumstance is to recognize an impending failure and correct it before it interferes with instrument function. A power switch may still be operative, but has lost its distinctive "click" and its solid "feel" when thrown. A cable may still work, but the insulation is cracked. A power plug may work but clearly mates improperly into its socket. It is advised to replace these defective but still-operative components.

It is also worthwhile to anticipate the consumption of some supplies such as ink or paper. If these supplies are not expensive, and if interruption of the measurements to replace these supplies would be adverse, it may be beneficial to replenish the supply within the instrument even if it means discarding some small remainder.

It is not necessary to routinely replace parts that are working appropriately. As mentioned above, the time and place of component failure is frequently unpredictable, and there is the possibility of inadvertently causing damage during a repair. Some parts, especially mechanical components, do have a well-established lifespan. For example, industrial equipment containing mechanical parts sometimes has timers or frequency counters that keep track of the amount of time or effort expended by the machine. However, very few laboratory instruments have such a precisely known lifespan. If predictable maintenance and replacement events are known for a piece of equipment, it may be advisable to maintain a use-log, or to install a timing or use device.

Reference Laboratory.—Instrument malfunction can be subtle, especially when calibration standards are not readily available or when instrument failure is not manifested in a gross way. Reference laboratory services have been established to assist laboratories in the maintenance of instruments used for biochemical measurements. These laboratories usually supply the investigator with an unknown sample or set of unknown samples, and then evaluate the result obtained by the investigator. They should be considered as part of maintenance under special and well-defined circumstances.

Repair and Troubleshooting

A Few Golden Rules.—At the outset, it is important to mention a few rules that bear on this area.

Don't panic. Most broken equipment isn't broken, but rather misconnected or maladapted. Panic tends to invade the brain of the novice scientist about the time that data are to be collected, or the boss is watching, and the instrument doesn't work. Panic is especially pernicious because it clouds a careful approach to equipment malfunction; because it leads to unnecessary attempted repairs; because it potentially worsens the failure; and because it may lead to hazardous approaches to repair or application.

Don't do more than you understand. Taking the cover off of a chassis labeled "no user serviceable parts" is not going to be productive. Wisdom is the better part of valor, and your local instrumentation department is unlikely to be appreciative of missing hold-down bolts or disconnected wires.

Don't expose yourself to an electrical or mechanical hazard. Keep yourself and items attached to you (watches, rings, ties) clear of moving hazards. Be cautious when working with line (115 VAC) electrical power, and be cautious of working with the output of high voltage power supplies. A good rule of thumb is, when first approaching the interior of an instrument whose exact layout is unknown, only work with one hand, while keeping the other hand in your pocket. This is an attempt to avoid a grounded pathway for the flow of current through your body. In this regard, battery-operated instruments, unless powered by high-voltage batteries, are considerably safer than line-operated instruments.

Goals of Troubleshooting.—Your goals are (1) to ascertain that a bona fide problem exists; (2) to be able to describe the mode of failure of the instrument, including the events or circumstances leading up to the failure; (3) to know what is correctable by you, and what must be turned over to others; and (4) to consider whether equipment failure, especially when repeated or catastrophic, offers the opportunity to replace rather than to repair equipment. With these goals in mind, let's examine some common modes of equipment failure.

Instrument Dead—Power Does not Come on.—Knowledge of the pathway of power to the instrument is the key to this usually correctable event (Fig 10–1). Power is usually supplied from a line source (the wall outlet), sometimes from batteries, or rarely from both. It passes into a mating plug, through a cord, and into a switch. In series with the instrument side of the switch is a fuse. In parallel with the instrument side of the switch may be a power indicator light or meter.

1. Line voltage is supplied to the instrument through the typical 115 VAC supply, which has a three-hole wall outlet and matching three-blade plug at the end of the power cord. Some pieces of equipment containing heavy duty motors or large heating elements may require 220 volt power, which is distinguished by a different configuration in which all the blades of the power cord are angled at 120° from each other. Outlets and instrument power plug connectors must mate properly—don't be foolish and attempt to mate two dissimilar plugs. Inspect the electrical plug to see if it is intact and to check the integrity of the wire running to the plug. Molded plugs that entirely encase the wire in opaque material are noninspectable. All new equipment should come with a hospital-grade plug (see chapter 7, Fig 7–3), which reduces the tension of the wire in the cord as it enters the plug and, if it is clear, allows observation of obvious wire breaks or disconnections within the plug.

2. Check that power is present at the wall outlet. Check that the outlet is live with the proper voltmeter, or plug in another instrument or electrical device that is known to work and check its operation. If it doesn't, the wall outlet may be defective, or the circuit breaker feeding the outlet may have tripped. Sometimes, power is fed to a local distribution strip into which the instrument is plugged. This strip may have its own switch and circuit breaker. Make sure the switch is on and the

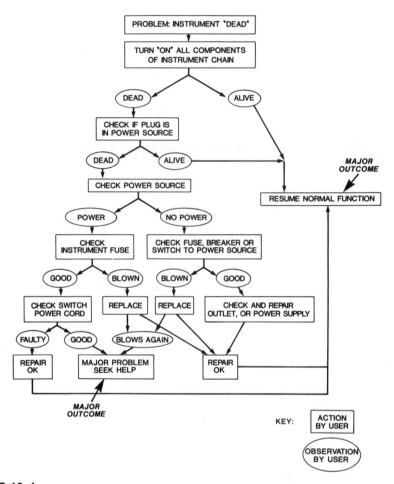

FIG 10–1.
Algorithm for problem solving—"dead" instrument. The user sequentially observes and acts to determine the cause of the problem. There are two major outcomes: either normal function resumes, or it is determined that there is a major problem for which the user should seek help.

breaker is reset. With the help of building maintenance people, locate and correct the problem. If power is available at the outlet, and the plug appears to be in order, follow the wire as it enters the case of the instrument to observe for breaks or failure of the wire.

3. Check the fuse or its equivalent, the circuit breaker. These devices act as a safety relief valve that fails or trips if overloaded. Some

fuseholders or circuit breakers are placed externally on the case. The circuit breaker, if tripped, simply can be reset. The fuse will require removal and replacement. Sometimes, these devices are placed within the instrument case, and removal and inspection require disassembly of the case. You must remove power from the instrument (unplug it) before removing the case. Glass-encased "buss" fuses are the most common variety of instrument fuse (Fig 10–2). All instruments that operate on line power will be fused immediately after the line cord enters the case. Fuses are rated by the current they can carry before failing (e.g., 1 amp), and by the time latency until they fail at current overload ("blow")—either normal (rapid) or time-delay ("slow blow"). The current rating of the fuse is matched to that of the instrument, and is based on the capacity of one or more components of the instrument to carry a current load that results in abnormal heating and therefore malfunction or damage to the component. A time-delay fuse is used for instruments that have a higher, but temporary, current at the time they are switched on (in-rush current) than the normal operating current. For example, instruments that contain a power supply (a component of many instruments) require a higher in-rush current than steady-state current at the time they are switched on to allow for the charging of large capacitors that are part of the power supply. Fuses without time delay are used for all other purposes. There may be more than one fuse and more than one fuse type within an instrument. For example,

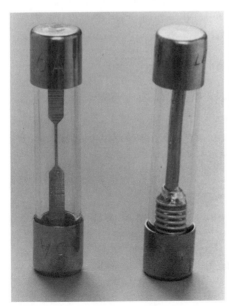

FIG 10–2.
Glass instrument fuses. Fuses are rated by the maximum current flow and by the duration of the current flow before failure. The rating is finely etched on the metal caps at the end of the fuse. The thin filament in the fuse at left indicates a fuse that blows rapidly after current overload. This type of fuse is used in most applications. The thick and spiral filament of the fuse at right is used in a fuse that responds slowly to current overload. This type of fuse is usually reserved for large instrument power supplies. A fuse should be used that conforms with the instrument manufacturer's printed specification. The specification may be embossed on the instrument case or published in the instrument manual.

a power supply may contain more than one fuse: one on the line input side, and one of the conditioned output side. The repair manual and schematic will identify their location and type.

A glass fuse can be visually inspected for failure, or tested by a resistance (ohm) meter: its metallic filament should be intact and its electrical properties should be "closed" (in continuity) and show negligible resistance. Ceramic fuses cannot be inspected visually and require testing. If the fuse is "open," or if in doubt, replace the fuse with the same rating and type specified by the schematics or identified on the fuse and check operation of the instrument.

Why did the fuse blow? Fuses are essentially mechanical devices with a limited lifespan that will eventually wear out and fail. However, observe the following precautions. If there was evidence of a burning smell, vaporization of instrument components, or repeated failure of the replacement fuse, do not continue operation without a complete instrumentation check. The fuse was there for a safety purpose.

4. Power indicators (either a light or a meter), which are used to inform the user that power is reaching the instrument, are in themselves subject to failure. If only the power light ("idiot" light) or meter has failed, the instrument will still receive power and function normally; otherwise, consider a switch failure.

5. At this point, remove the power plug from the wall as you investigate further. The switch should be checked for proper operation. Sometimes the switch can be accessed directly by unscrewing it from the chassis; most of the time, the case has to be more completely disassembled. All the wires intended for the switch should be attached securely or soldered to it. When continuity is checked by a resistance meter, the switch should show an electrical "open" and a "close" between its contacts (there may be more than one set) when toggled back and forth between off and on, respectively.

6. If these checks do not successfully remedy the problem—line power, wall outlet and instrument plug and cord, fuse, power display, and instrument switch—go no further without consulting qualified repair personnel.

Power On, but No Signal Output.—Knowledge of the pathway of the flow of signal through the instrumentation chain is critical to the correct diagnosis of this problem (Fig 10–3). This flow has been described in detail in chapters 4 through 9. Here, it is only necessary to review the hardware considerations briefly. Instrumentation usually

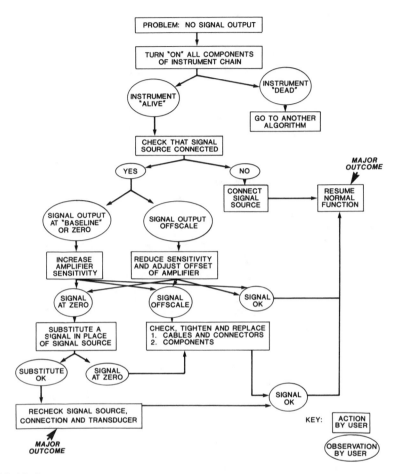

FIG 10–3.
Algorithm for problem solving—no signal output. The user sequentially observes and acts to determine the cause of the problem. There are two major outcomes: either normal function resumes, or the actual source of the signal needs to be verified.

implies (at a minimum) a transducer, an amplifier, and a display device. Sometimes, the hardware devices are identifiable as single devices, but frequently they are packaged together or bundled. For diagnostic purposes, it is important to break a bundled device apart in order to localize the problem.

1. Check to make sure that the power has been turned on to *all* of the instruments; sometimes, a single power supply feeds multiple de-

vices within a chassis, and although the main power supply may be operative, the individual devices may not be switched on.

2. Check to see that signal is going into and out of the instruments. The hookup from the source of the signal into the device may not have been completed, or may have failed. Edge connectors between printed circuit boards and instrument chassis can work themselves loose. Also, edge connectors may not provide good electrical contact if they become oxidized or if they accumulate foreign substances (such as skin oils from inadvertent touching). Clean the edge connector with a rubber eraser or special cleaning compound and reinsert securely. Cables can cause some vexing problems. Once the instrumentation chain has been assembled, label the cables with what type of signal they are carrying, and which end goes into which instrument. Paper gummed labels, further secured by transparent tape to the cable, are very good for this purpose. Look for obviously broken or inadequately connected cables. Cables frequently terminate in connectors that require special care and attention to mating of plug and jack. The connector may not have been pushed fully "home." If in doubt, swap out connecting cables with ones that are known to work. Destroy or throw away cables that don't work or are doubtful, lest they be reused accidentally. That piece of advice alone is worth the purchase price of this book.

3. Inject a known signal into the front end of the system. If the system uses a pressure transducer, pressurize that transducer with a known pressure source, such as a mercury manometer. If no signal appears, the individual components of the system will have to be checked. A signal may appear, but may be unsatisfactory because of calibration or some other problem. This type of check is best performed with a signal simulator, which injects signals of known energy type, amplitude, and frequency content. Instrument repair specialists have access to this type of equipment.

4. Take the system apart instrument by instrument and replace each component of the system. Transducers are especially likely to break since they are intended to be sensitive devices that are handled repetitively. Replace the current transducer with one that is known to be working. A good rule of thumb is to replace everything twice (if needed), because of the slim-but-real chance of coming across two consecutive nonworking components.

5. Sometimes the failure mode of a transducer or other instrument results in a fixed but bizarre output. Check the reading reported by the

display device and consult the operations manual of the instrument in question to determine if this is this level represents a message that indicates failure.

6. If the display device has failed, two recommended devices may be substituted. The superior device, but one less readily available, is an oscilloscope. This allows one to see the dynamic output of the signal and, because it can be calibrated, to determine whether the signal amplitude is as expected. A device that is almost as good is the voltmeter part of the VOM, especially if it is a digital voltmeter (DVM). Although one cannot observe the dynamic aspects of the signal, the polarity and amplitude of the signal are frequently sufficient to determine the operation of the instrument up to the display device. In fact, as mentioned in chapter 9, a DVM is highly recommended to assist in calibration before running the experiment.

Intermittent Failure.—I have saved for the final point of discussion the intermittent failure, which is the most vexing of all equipment malfunctions. Typically, an intermittent failure will occur as follows. The instrumentation power-up and calibration proceeds normally. In the middle of the data collection, the display device records no signal output, or paroxysmally records a signal output. The intermittent failure is especially pernicious, because it destroys the user's confidence in the instrument, and frequently frustrates rapid repair, even by highly qualified personnel. Two common causes of intermittent failures are faulty cables and connectors, and failed components that are susceptible to normal heating as instrument operation proceeds from a cold start to steady-state temperature.

1. Sometimes it's just not possible to explain why a cable or connector causes an intermittent failure. They should be high on your list of possibilities, and they should be systematically replaced and tightened.

2. Failed components, which operated until a critical thermal point was reached, may be difficult to identify. Carefully note the time from power-on until the time of failure and the circumstances of the experiment that surrounded the failure. At the time of the failure, be prepared to quickly swap out components in the system with the possibility of at least localizing the problem. Where a thermal failure of an electronic component is suspected, an aerosolized form of refrigerant can be sprayed on individual components to cause cool-down and to observe for return of proper operation.

Noise and Interference.—This is dealt with in chapter 9 as part of setting up and running the equipment. Here, under instrument repair, it is worth mentioning that instrument failure can be manifested as noise. This is especially true for cables and amplifiers. Capacitors, which are included as components in many instruments, eventually deteriorate and leak their dielectric (usually silicone oil). This may be marked by the sudden appearance of an enormous amount of noise.

11

Obtaining or Purchasing Instruments

The material presented so far presumes that the scientist already has instruments; this may not be so. In this chapter we will explore the mechanisms available to the novice investigator for obtaining or purchasing instruments, and for evaluating instruments before purchase.

WHAT YOU NEED TO KNOW

1. Review your needs for instrumentation. You may not need to obtain an additional instrument. What you or a colleague already have on hand could very well be sufficient.

2. Research the characteristics and sources of instruments that are appropriate and available for your study.

3. It is far better to "beg, borrow, or steal" a piece of equipment, than to purchase some equipment.

4. Regardless of the source from which the equipment is obtained, you must be able to identify and evaluate the specifications of the equipment.

5. You may have to run the administrative gauntlet of obtaining funds and making the administrative arrangements to purchase equipment.

Do You Need an Additional Instrument?

In chapter 2, I pointed out that understanding the characteristics of the signal to be measured will determine whether you need an instrument, and will suggest the specifications of the instrument to be used. In chapter 4, I went so far as to suggest that sometimes you don't even need an instrument. Because of the rapidity—and evanescence—with which science is conducted, expending time and effort in obtaining funds and approval for an instrument, and waiting around for the instrument to arrive, may not be productive. That is, you may decide to make do with what you already have. This advice is not given lightly. Anyone who has to deal with the bureaucratic machinery for obtaining an instrument will quickly evaluate whether or not this is the route to go.

Frequently, a colleague has an instrument in place and in good working order that you can use for your experiment. You may have to move the location of your experiment to that other laboratory, or you may decide to bring samples or specimens to that laboratory. Once you have made the decision to actually own or be in charge of instruments, you have also made additional decisions to properly operate, maintain, and potentially loan out those instruments—additional demanding obligations that come with the territory.

Gather Background Information

In general, knowledge of instruments grows monotonically with your duration and expertise in a particular field. But everyone has to start somewhere. You need sources of information about instruments, and you need to understand the principles of operation and the construction of instruments.

Sources of Information About Instruments
A wide variety of sources is available from which to assemble comprehensive information on what instrument is best for your purposes.

Colleagues.—Your colleagues will frequently have, or will be aware of, types of instruments, or manufacturers from which to obtain information.

Research Publications.—The "methods" sections of papers that investigate the same phenomena in which you are interested should describe in detail the types and the application of instruments appropriate to the experiments. In addition to a description of the function of an instrument in a particular experiment, the paper may reference additional scientific papers that provide detailed explanations and technical evaluations of the instrument. The model number and name of the manufacturer should be included in the publication.

Conventions and Trade Shows.—Scientific conventions and trade shows will frequently assemble a large number of manufacturers and distributors for the convenience and interest of conference registrants. Such shows are frequently beneficial to a potential customer, because the instrument manufacturers may have the instruments on hand for inspection and demonstration, and because a wide variety of knowledgeable personnel may be available to answer questions. This is a good excuse to get your boss to pay for a trip. The management of a convention or trade show will frequently publish a catalog indexed by both manufacturer and type of instrument, which will assist you in focusing on your particular needs. Because of the wide variety of instrumentation displayed, some annual conventions can be especially recommended (Table 11–1); these should not be considered to the exclusion of other shows conducted by subspecialty societies and professional organizations.

Advertising.—Advertisements in journals and publications will often call your attention to a particular manufacturer or device.

Sales Representatives.—Manufacturers, distributors, and salespeople are widely available to provide advice, mail literature, and demonstrate instruments. These people make their living this way, and should be very receptive to assisting you in your questions. Be wary of the promissory note that advertises the near-availability of an instrument; the latency between prototype and commercial model is unpredictable.

Consultants.—Someone once defined a consultant as "a person who asks to borrow your watch and then tells you the time." The implication, perhaps true, is that you already have all the information at your disposal and that an additional opinion is not needed. However, emerging and sophisticated technology may have important nuances that take a large amount of time and effort to master. At present, com-

TABLE 11–1.
Annual Conventions That Have Major Displays of Instruments

NAME OF ORGANIZATION	ADDRESS OF ORGANIZATION
American Association for the Advancement of Science (AAAS)	1333 H Street NW Washington, DC 20005
American Association of Medical Instrumentation (AAMI)	1901 N Ft Myer Dr Suite 602 Arlington, VA 22209
Federation of American Societies for Experimental Biology (FASEB)	9650 Rockville Pike Bethesda, MD 20814

COMPENDIA OF SCIENTIFIC INSTRUMENTS AND LITERATURE	
NAME OF SOURCE	ADDRESS OF SOURCE
Annual Guide to Scientific Instruments (Publication)	American Association for the Advancement of Science 1333 H Street NW Washington, DC 20005
Biomedical Engineering Decision Support Services (Computerized product and technical literature)	BMEDSS Department Akron City Hospital 525 East Market St Akron, OH 44309

puter technology best exemplifies this parameter. Under special circumstances a consultant can be recommended to assist in the selection of instruments.

Compendia.—Some journals and professional organizations publish directories of instruments and instrument manufacturers as a service to their membership, and a computerized product and technical literature service is available by phone link (see Table 11–1).

Principles of Operation and Construction
There is a hierarchical plane of concepts on which instruments are built. One plane is the basic physical, mechanical, and electronic principles of the instrumentation. It is certainly helpful to have a grasp of these. The second plane of organization is the actual construction or assembly of the instrumentation.

Basic Principles of Operation.—It is quite useful to have a grasp of the physical and biologic principles on which biomedical instruments are based. Uncover your long-forgotten elementary physics, chemistry, electronics, and mathematics books and spend some time reviewing this material.

It is also very important that you understand the principles of the method of measurement of the instrument. This is an absolutely crucial piece of background information. Failure to carry out this step frequently results in less-than-optimal instrumentation and experimental design. To accomplish this, you need to recognize the type and energy content of the signal to be measured (see chapter 2), and the physical principle by which this signal can be detected—its transducible property (chapter 5). For certain signals, this problem collapses to a single possibility. For example, an electrical signal of muscle, nerve, or heart requires the appropriate electrode and an amplifier that are capable of detecting and amplifying electrical activity; it is then only necessary to match the equipment's specifications with the properties of the signal.

However, some other signals may be detected in a variety of ways, and a preference among the choices may be ambiguous. For example, oxygen concentration of blood or fluids may be measured by a biochemical electrode (oxygen tension), by spectrophotometry (oxygen saturation), or by fuel cell (oxygen content). Each of these instruments may be satisfactory, or perhaps none will. As another example, cardiac wall motion or mass may be measured by imaging techniques that use x-rays, ultrasound, radionuclides, or nuclear magnetic resonance imaging. The actual principles of detection are different, and offer the investigator a number of choices and options. Therefore, information should be obtained about the actual physical principle involved in the detection of the signal.

The most pressing need, and the most important recent advance in biomedical instrumentation, has been the development of new signal detectors. When new principles of detection are discovered, they quickly will be published in journals and other technical sources, unless they have proprietary value to a manufacturer. As the information becomes more formalized, books and symposia will appear. As the principles are translated into instruments that are used for measurements, publications by authors who have used these instruments will appear. These papers should include an adequate "methods" section, or refer to prior publications or technical bulletins that will inform the reader about the principles and application of the instruments. The scientist should be aware of all the possibilities for signal detection before making a decision as to which instrumentation to use. If no satisfactory principle of detection is yet available, it offers the challenge and the opportunity to invent your own!

Construction and Packaging of the Instrument.—The physical and biologic principles governing the operation of an instrument are concretized into the actual instrument form. A manufacturer packages these principles into one of two forms: either a completed instrument suitable for purchase by an end user, or an incomplete form that is bought by some other manufacturer and completed into a product. This latter form is called OEM, or original equipment of manufacture.

Most users are aware only of a finished product and not the OEM form because they only see advertised and demonstrated products that are the complete form. Some manufacturers can produce multiple components of a complicated instrument and are capable of integrating these into a completed instrument. They profit from the ability to both manufacture and sell a completed instrument to the retail market. The user pays a high price for a completed product that is ready for off-the-shelf use, supported by a cadre of sales and service representatives.

Users are less aware that some manufacturers of instruments, such as recorders, are not capable of or interested in the final packaging of an instrument or in its sales to a retail customer. They produce components that other manufacturers purchase and incorporate into a completed instrument and that they modify and prepare for the end user. This type of instrument is called OEM.

It is possible for the user to purchase not only completed instruments, but frequently OEM components. The latter may have to be modified and adapted for use, and frequently are not accompanied by a sales force or field service. However, the user has considerable flexibility in the adaptation of these components, and saves a considerable amount of money in their purchase.

Borrowing, Begging, or Stealing

There are excellent reasons for not buying a piece of equipment, and some opportunities to avoid doing so. The vast percentage of money available for research is used for the salaries of personnel and, to some extent, for supplies. This is as it should be, because people and ideas make experiments, assisted by machines. Institutions and grants only grudgingly make monies available for major equipment purchases, and there usually are substantial requirements necessary for this justification (more about that later). There are a number of opportunities to obtain equipment that both avoid the process of applying for funds for instrumentation and keep whatever limited bucks you have available reserved for what makes your experiment run.

The most important aspect of using this avenue, which avoids instrument purchase, is the maintenance of good personal contact with a number of people who have access to instruments. And so, this very technical book is now reduced to a lesson in maintaining excellent personal relationships. In addition to your colleagues, administrator, department head, and dean, it is important to get to know instrument representatives and salesmen. Providing them with a very small amount of your valuable time will reap large rewards when you need their help.

When you borrow equipment, it is imperative that you maintain and return it in good working order; you will never get a second loan from someone to whom you return (and do not inform about) a non-working piece of equipment.

Borrowing Instruments From Colleagues

Why would you want to borrow equipment? Not only does it preserve resources, it also allows one to stay current with the advances in instrumentation. If you have finally convinced the dean or the study section to let you buy equipment, you're then stuck with using that equipment. If you haven't yet used up that perquisite, you can reserve it for the next round of instrumentation advances. This concept is very topical, since many forms of instruments that recently were upgraded by the inclusion of integrated circuit design are again in the process of upgrade through the addition of microprocessor (computer) components. Don't invest your effort and money and then be stuck with less-than-optimal equipment.

Large departments usually contain a large amount of instrumentation, and frequently generate a good deal of older but still operational equipment. It is likely that what you need already exists close at hand, and it is ego, or lack of a friendly relationship, that prevents the usage of such equipment. Intradepartmental loans of equipment are far more common than interdepartmental or interinstitutional; however, everything is possible.* Before you borrow a piece of equipment, make sure it meets your specifications, with respect to experimental design and technical aspects. When you borrow the equipment, *make sure to also borrow the operations and the repair manuals.*

Begging Instruments From Manufacturers (Donations)

Under some circumstances, equipment manufacturers will loan an investigator an instrument—either temporarily or permanently. It is very common to allow an investigator to evaluate a piece of equipment

---

*Witness the cell separator and other instruments and medical devices the UCLA School of Medicine loaned to the Soviet Union for assistance in bone marrow transplantation after the Chernobyl nuclear power plant accident in the spring of 1986.

for a varying length of time in the laboratory. This may impose an unwritten obligation to buy the instrument if it proves satisfactory, but manufacturers and their representatives expect that a large number of times a purchase will not occur.

An even more satisfactory arrangement can be made in the evaluation of new or prototype instruments, where the manufacturer is attempting to achieve an entry into the marketplace. Instruments are frequently given to important or notable laboratories for the sole purpose of obtaining their comments, and for the hope that the good experience of that laboratory will be transmitted to colleagues, which ultimately will result in sales.

Some institutions and departments purchase such a large amount of instruments from a particular manufacturer, or maintain such good relationships, that they are willing to loan a piece of equipment to a department.

"Steal" Equipment

Although the actual illegal act of stealing cannot be condoned, there are some circumstances in which taking matters into your own hands may be effective. Equipment is frequently abandoned or placed in storage, only to be forgotten or unused. Snooping around with your equipment manager or querying your colleagues will sometimes uncover such equipment. It is always advisable to obtain the permission of the owner before usage.

Be wary of equipment for which manuals and schematics are not available and the specifications are unknown. Although it may be possible to calibrate the instrument and determine its specifications, it is very difficult to reconstruct information on operation, maintenance, and repair. Additionally, an instrument may be crippled to the point of nonusage because parts that are vital to the operation of the instrument are no longer available. This is especially true for copies of software that have been obtained illegally—"pirated" software. Such software is frequently useless, either because the copy is inadequte or because the original documentation that accompanied the software is not available.

Evaluating Equipment Under Loan

It may be assumed appropriately that new equipment meets the manufacturer's written specifications. It is inappropriate to make such an assumption for used or borrowed equipment. It is important to check the following.

Safety.—Electrical safety standards and methodology have advanced rapidly (see chapter 1). Older or used equipment may not be current, or may have accumulated a defect. Have your instrumentation repair and maintenance department assist you in evaluating the electrical safety of the equipment.

Inspect the electrical outlet cord; most older cords were made of hard rubber that cracked with use and age, and were not equipped with hospital-grade plugs. Fittings and connectors may have worn and require repair or replacement. Evaluate for current leakage. Many older pieces of equipment do not meet specifications for current leakage. Be wary of using such equipment for human connection. Frequently, such equipment can be made safe by the installation of an isolation transformer, which will cost a pretty penny, but may only be a small percentage of the cost of a new instrument.

Performance.—Operating characteristics of the used eqiupment may have deviated from the original specifications. Before collecting data, make sure that the equipment is in proper working order and evaluate accuracy, precision, resolution, range, hysteresis, and frequency response (see chapter 3).

Analog Equipment Specifications

It is absolutely vital that you obtain and evaluate equipment specifications. Do not purchase any equipment unless the specifications have been made available and have been reviewed. There is no such thing as "specifications aren't available," or "specifications cannot be easily obtained." Also, do not assume a particular specification. If it is not supplied, it is either not known or doesn't exist. There are two broad categories of equipment specification: environmental operating conditions, and specifications of signal processing.

Operating Conditions

All instruments have been evaluated to operate under specified conditions (Table 11–2). Except for instruments that do not require any source of power (such as an electrode), the source of the power will be explicitly stated: 110 or 220 VAC and, for instruments with motors, single- or three-phase; or battery operation or equipped for foreign country electrical power or DC operation. For electronic equipment, an issue of concern is that of range of ambient temperature. This will usually be stated as "operating temperatures from 'x' to 'y' degrees." An

TABLE 11–2.

Operating Conditions

PARAMETER	SPECIFICATION
Electrical power	
Source	AC, DC, battery
Quantity	Phase, voltage, current, power
Environment	
Temperature	Temperature range
Humidity	Humidity range
Position mounted	Any, horizontal, vertical
Vibration	
Transportable	Yes, no, maybe
Impact	g-forces, impact forces
Special characteristics	Should be fully described

operating range for relative humidity may also be included in the specifications. Vibration specification, particularly for instruments that are expected to be portable, may be important for equipment containing delicate electronic or mechanical components. This may be stated as, "will withstand 'x' g-forces" or "will withstand 'y' force of component 'a' striking component 'b'." Some instruments may have exotic or unusual specifications of operating environment. Contrariwise, your intended usage may be different from that for which the instrument was designed such as unusual humidity, dust, radiation, or explosive environments. Do not assume that an instrument can be adapted to an unusual or harsh operating environment without assurance from the manufacturer.

Signal Processing
These specify the operations you want the instrument to perform. The qualities have been mentioned in chapter 3, and are only repeated here for convenience with reference to an example specification sheet.

Type of Instrument.—The function and application of the instrument. This is reported as a single function (e.g., transducer, amplifier, or recorder, etc.) or a series of components intended for multiple functions (e.g., amplifier and CRT display and photographic recorder).

Accuracy.—The ability to detect exact quantities. This is usually reported as a percentage of the range of the instrument, or as an absolute quantity, or both.

Precision.—The ability to reproduce quantitative measurement. This is usually reported as a percentage of the range of the instrument or as an absolute quantity, or both.

Range.—The scale over which the quantity can be measured. This is expressed in absolute units of the measurement.

Resolution.—The resolving power to which the quantity will be reported. This is reported either as a percentage of the scale or in absolute quantities.

Linearity and Hysteresis.—The ability to maintain precision over the range of operation or in absolute units.

Frequency Response and Rise Time.—The frequency characteristics of the instrument. For many instruments, frequency response is reported at the 3 dB (decreased to 0.707) of the flat portion of the bandwidth. For some instruments, bandwidth may be reported at some other value, such as 0.5 dB or perhaps 0.95 dB. Rise time, which is an approximation of the high-frequency cutoff (see chapter 2), is sometimes reported in lieu of bandwidth. This is the time it takes an instrument to achieve a certain fraction of a step change in signal level, such as 0.95 or 0.90 of the final signal level.

Input and Output Impedence.—When amplifiers are included as part of the instrument, this specifies the electrical transfer characteristics of signals coming into the instrument and signals leaving the instrument.

Gain.—This specifies the maximum or the range of multiplication as a dimensionless ratio or the ratio of output/input.

Offset, Drift, and Noise.—The amount of nonrandom and random error caused by the instrument. The level of these errors is frequently specified for certain operating conditions, such as temperature. Usually expressed as a percentage or as an absolute quantity of the signal under study.

Electrical Safety.—This provides either an absolute number of the leakage current of the case to ground, or indicates conformance with some safety standard, or indicates actual approval by some inspection authority as having conformed with a safety standard of a recognized authority.

Warranty.—What the manufacturer/distributor expressly implies as to the warranty of the equipment. This may or may not include information concerning compliance with local regulations governing warranties including information about implied warranty.

Example of Simple Instrument Specifications
It is instructive to examine the specifications of one of the simplest instruments available—an electrode (Table 11–3).

Description.—This provides a minimum classification of what type of instrument is specified. In these specifications, we are dealing with a skin electrode. "Fixed lead" implies that the electrode has a permanent lead wire attached to it that will connect to another cable or amplifier. Some literature doesn't give the reader the courtesy of instru-

---

TABLE 11–3.

Example of Electrode Specifications

Description
  Fixed lead biopotential skin electrode
Applications
  Clear and stable transmission of ECG, EEG, EMG, ENG, EOG, and other skin
    biopotentials; ideal for routine clinical monitoring and for research studies.
Construction
  Sensor
    1 mm thick sintered silver/silver chloride. Available in 4-, 8-, and 12.5-mm
      diameters. Corresponding housing for sensor is 7.2, 12.5, and 16.5 mm,
      respectively
  Lead
    PVC insulated lead wire of copper conductor wrapped terminating in standard
      2-mm diameter silver-plated pin. Available in 60 and 100 cm lengths
Electrical specifications*
  DC offset voltage: 180 μV
  Drift: 25 μV/h (at constant temperature)
  Noise: 1 μV peak-to-peak
  Polarization: 2 to 4 μV at 0.1 μamp
Connection to signal source
  Electrodes can be attached to the skin with inexpensive adhesive washers, tape, or
    retention bands
Connection to other instruments
  Compatible with most recording and monitoring systems

---

*After prolonged soaking in 0.9% saline. Median values from a large sample.

ment classification. It provides a trade name and a glossy picture and assumes we know what it is we're about to read.

Applications.—This informs us that this skin electrode could be useful for recording any one of a number of biopotentials from the skin surface. The terms "clear and stable" are gratuitous. Would they sell us an electrode that didn't provide suitable signals?

Construction.—The sensor itself is made of the typical and preferred material, silver/silver chloride. The size of the electrode and housing will be a determinant of the skin sites and conditions to which we can apply the electrode. The lead wire terminates in standard pin configuration. This means it should fit the standard cable that connects skin electrodes to an amplifier.

Electrical Specifications.—Four electrical specifications are shown. These are actually error specifications. The footnote indicates under what conditions they were obtained, and indicates that this represents an average performance. We have previously discussed offset, drift, and noise (see chapters 3 and 9). Notice the large bias that is typical for an electrode and that necessitates an AC-coupled amplifier. Here, an additional specification is supplied. Polarization is the opposing voltage (back voltage) generated in the system by a signal of specified current.

Connection to Signal Source.—Note that this surface electrode requires some fastening material in order for it to adhere to the skin.

Connection to Other Instruments.—We are given some assurance that this instrument will work with most other devices. Other than a nonstandard pin on the electrode lead, surface electrodes should be compatible with other instruments, and we are left wondering exactly what incompatibilities there could be.

Example of More Complex Instrument Specifications
As another example, let's review the specifications for a multichannel physiologic recording instrument (Table 11–4).

Description.—This is a six-channel instrument (see limitations described below) that houses physiologic amplifiers, a display, and a recorder.

TABLE 11–4.

Example of Recording System Specification

Description
Six-channel signal conditioner, display, and recording system
Application
Physiologic data acquisition
Power requirement
105–130 V or 210–260 V AC, 50–60 Hz, single phase
Physical dimensions
Overall size of cabinet is 145 cm H, 61 cm W, 82 cm D
Net weight is 125 kg; shipping weight is 148 kg
Temperature range
Operating temperature from 10°C to 40°C
Storage temperature from −10°C to 60°C
Display screen
CRT phosphor type, six-channel display, 30 cm width
Sweep speeds from 5 to 500 mm/sec
Recorder
Photographic recorder with frequency response of 0–5,000 Hz
Printer width of 18 cm. Accepts 60-m rolls. Three paper/developer choices
Speeds from 5 to 500 mm/sec
Channel spaces
Maximum of six signal conditioners; amplifiers available for ECG, pressure, phonocardiography, respiration, echocardiography and DC; a variety of signal processors and interfaces to tape and computer systems
Electrical safety
Chassis leakage: <100 μamp
Isolated patient plug-ins: <10 μamp
Meets or surpasses all safety requirements of present standards

Electrical Requirements.—The instrument is adaptable to the usual forms of available line power.

Physical Dimensions.—The height (H), width (W), and depth (D) are shown. The shipping weight would include packaging material to ensure safety during transport. This could make a difference in determining shipping charges or for making provision of movement of the instrument when it arrives on location.

Operating Range.—Two ranges are shown: the operating range and the storage range.

Monitor.—This is a cathode ray tube (CRT) monitor that is 30 cm wide. We are not told how high it is. (I couldn't determine this anywhere in the literature—a picture suggested that it was a little less high than it was wide). The screen is coated with a phosphor, which should allow some persistence until overwritten on the next flyback, but the duration of the persistance was not quoted. The sweep speeds would show a screen duration of from 0.6 seconds to 60 seconds (30 cm/times sweep speed). No specification is provided for frequency response: we assume it is some large number of kHz, but we may want to know this for sure.

Recorder.—This is a photographic recorder that has a typically wide bandwidth. Note the relatively narrow paper width in response to paper expense. Roles of paper are 60 m long, and there are some options in the paper type and the developing process. A range of recording speeds is provided.

Channels.—There is a wide variety of signal conditioners available for the instrument, and a maximum of six can be accommodated. However, some of the widely used amplifiers are "double high," and these would occupy the chassis space of two conditioners and thereby reduce the total number of channels. Signal processors (such as a differentiator/integrator) and interface devices (such as to a tape recorder) would further reduce the number of available amplifier channels.

Electrical Safety.—The case of the instrument leaks to ground a maximum of 100 microamps. Isolation systems in each signal conditioner which has a lead wire or attachment to the patient limits leakage current to ground of 10 μamp. We are told the instrument meets all safety standards, but we are not told to which safety standards this refers.

Computer Hardware and Software

Although all the general information, rules, and advice that apply to analog instrumentation apply to digital instrumentation, there are some additional considerations. These are the relationship between the software (the instructions used to program the computer) and the hardware (the physical components that execute the software). Although both need to be considered when a computer system purchase is at hand, it is very clear that *primary consideration should be given to the software.* Once the proper software is chosen, one then picks the hardware that is required to execute the software.

How Do You Know You Need a Computer?

The most compelling reason for obtaining a computer system is to have a definite task—an application—in mind. Although a general knowledge of computers can be lauded as an educational effort, it will be a vacant exercise without an application. With a computer system, the investigator must be prepared to devote a very large amount of time at the beginning before anything useful will occur. Without a clear application in mind, the rewards intrinsic to "computer hacking" are just too small to warrant the time and effort.

In scientific computing, the usual applications are data acquisition and analysis (reviewed in chapter 8), database, statistical analysis, and word processing.

Software

The set of instructions that are executed by the hardware is called the software.

Software Types.—Software can be divided up into applications programs, productivity tools, and development tools. An applications program does as its name implies—it is applied to solve a particular problem. A productivity tool enhances the management of data, such as a spreadsheet or a statistical analysis package. A development tool is meant for a computer programmer—it is a computer language or similar program that assists in the writing of other computer programs.

The first two of these categories, applications programs and productivity tools, are what a scientist most often wants or needs. A development tool is reserved for that handful of scientists or laboratories who are developing their own software. Software development is unrealistic and not advised for most computer users except under unusual circumstances. Applications and productivity software will almost always be less expensive, easy and quickly set up and run, and more satisfactory to use than that which can be developed by nonprofessional programmers.

Evaluating Software.—A number of major and minor criteria are used to judge the quality of a software product (Table 11–5). The most obvious, but not necessarily the easiest to judge, is whether the software actually performs the task you want it to perform. Software is extremely focused in its execution, so that a near miss probably will be worthless to a computer user. The only way to know for sure is to try the software. Discussions with a colleague or a salesman, a demonstra-

TABLE 11–5.

Software Evaluation

Primary consideration
    Evaluation of software to fit a specific task
    Hardware availability and requirements
Secondary considerations
    Performance
    Error handling
    Ease of use
    Reliability
    Value for the money
    Documentation (written and during use)
Tertiary considerations
    Product support
    Copy protection
    Warranty

---

tion at a software showroom, and reading a product review and accompanying literature are all useful adjuncts. In that regard, it frequently makes sense to rely on an established product, especially if consideration is being given to the purchase of a productivity tool such as a word processor or spreadsheet, because the characteristics of the software are well known.

The other important principal criteria is the type and availability of hardware. The ramifications of this may range from the sublime to the ridiculous. A particular piece of software might be very apropos, but only suitable for a mainframe, whereas your budget, space, and computer support will only permit a microcomputer. Even within a class of computers, you should be aware that the software will be specific for one particular computer and for a minimum hardware configuration of that computer. For example, you would not want to buy software that required hardware that was not readily available. Also, you might want to reconsider a particular software program if it required special and expensive hardware.

There are other important issues that need to be addressed once it has been resolved that the software can perform the task required. These relate to the use of the program: performance, error handling, ease of use, reliability, value for the money, and documentation. The latter element—documentation—has proven to be an especially vexing problem. A product should be supported with complete and easy to understand written documentation, and the program should be supported during use with screen documentation. Note that price is only one of the considerations, and should be taken in the context of the others.

Still a third tier of considerations is issues of copy protection, product support, and warranty. The controversy over copy protection—the inability of a computer user to make additional copies of the software—continues to rage. If software is copy protected, it should either come with a backup copy or have excellent product support from the parent company so that a defective program can be exchanged rapidly for a working copy.

Pirated Software.—Copies of software that have been obtained without approval from a copyright source are consider to be pirated. The rights of the user and the rights of the copyright source aside, most of the software obtained this way is useless, either because the copy is inadequate or because there is no availability of documentation. For the user concerned about backup of a licensed or purchased program, the answer is to use only non–copy-protected software, or to use software from a source with superb product support.

Hardware

The physical components of the computer system that execute the instructions of the software are called the hardware.

Hardware Classification.—Computer hardware has been classified according to a number of factors into supercomputers, mainframes, minicomputers, and microcomputers or personal computers (see Table 8–1, chapter 8). The choice among these classes, and the specific computer chosen within a class, is almost entirely dependent on the application and the software chosen to execute the application. At the risk of enraging hardware manufacturers, there is virtual equality among computer systems within a particular class. Advertisements and salesmen are supposed to accentuate the small and usually less important nuances that distinguish one manufacturer's system from another. Indeed, at times there are important differences. But these differences are largely driven by *the availability of software for a particular computer system that will best accomplish your particular goals,* and not by the differences in hardware that will run the same software.

Hardware Specification.—*Identify the software to solve your problem or fulfill your application and then buy the hardware to support your software.* Part of the specifications for software is the required hardware. Software will specify for what computer system it is intended, and what components are necessary as a minimum and as an option.

For example, a word processor program would specify a particular computer system by computer class and, more specifically, by manufacturer (there may be more than one version of the program available for different classifications and manufacturers). The word processer program available for a microcomputer would require, as a minimum, the computer configured with a keyboard, some minimum amount of RAM, some form of mass storage such as a floppy disk, a monitor, and a printer. For optimum use of the program, which could make it easier or more efficient to use, or could make it possible to use all the "bells and whistles" of the program, additional hardware could include an advanced form of mass storage, a mouse, a graphics driver card and monitor, and a graphics printer.

As another example, a data acquisition program would specify a particular system by computer class and, more specifically, by manufacturer. The data acquisition system of a microcomputer would require, as a minimum, the computer configured with an analog-to-digital converter, some minimum amount of RAM, some form of mass storage device, and a graphics driver card and monochrome monitor. Options could include hardware such as a mouse and graphics printer, but could also include productivity software such as a spreadsheet and statistical package. These optional software tools are meant to work in concert with the original program in order to extend the analysis and presentation of the digitized data.

Running the Administrative Gauntlet

The final steps in equipment acquisition are obtaining the money and the act of purchasing and installing the instrument.

Getting the money

Whole books are written and courses given on grantsmanship. The reader is well advised to consult these resources. However, some recitals may be helpful. As indicated above, no source of money is wildly enthusiastic about the purchase of instruments. Perhaps because of the bias that they are expensive toys that are quickly outgrown and discarded ("the difference between men and boys is the price of their toys"), or perhaps because the bulk of money should flow to salaries and supplies, instrument purchase is given low priority. Agencies may explicitly state whether or not a grant can include a request for equipment, and they may state explicitly that the purpose of the grant is not to equip a laboratory. To cover for what they may consider a rare legitimate request, some agencies set aside specific monies and hold a specific competition for equipment. Given limited resources, the novice scientist may require the wisdom of Solomon on deciding among choices. *Documentation and careful justification* are the foundations to the success of obtaining money and approval for the purchase of instrumentation. The elements of a justification are as follows:

1. What do you need to measure, why do you need to measure that parameter, and why do you need an instrument to measure it?
2. Have you exhausted all possibilities to beg, borrow (or steal) an instrument? If allowed to purchase the instrument is there any evidence that it will be used for a long period, that it can be used for other experiments or other parameters so as to enhance its utility? Can it be shared in use to maximize its utility? Can it be shared in expense so as to spread the cost among multiple agencies and multiple investigators?
3. What are the exact specifications of the instrument? Do these specifications indicate the generic form of an instrument, or do they imply that only one manufacturer/model will suffice?
4. Have you obtained institutional approval to purchase, install, and use this equipment? Once in place, are there qualified personnel (specifically named in the application) to run and maintain the equipment? Who will repair the equipment, and do you have the money resources to pay for the repairs?

Getting Institutional Approval

Institutions have rigid and complex rules concerning equipment purchases. Let's look at it from their viewpoint: in addition to the same concerns of granting authorities, they also have to deal with the problems of space and installation, safety, and maintenance and repair. Woe to the investigator who has gone this far in the process of instrument acquisition, and hasn't gotten preliminary approval of the institution.

Earlier, we spoke about effective communication with other personnel, and that cannot be overemphasized. In each institution, there will be a group of personnel responsible for this area.

Department Administrator or Officer.—This is the first person to sign off on the purchase order. They need to know the same specifications that you would supply to a granting agency, and all the other information that's appropriate to the institution. They can be very helpful in dealing with the administrative bureaucracy.

Intermediate Approving Officer.—This person may be interposed in the purchase process to review some particular aspect of the situation, especially when large purchases are made, or especially if the institution finds itself bombarded by frequent requests for the same type of equipment which may be subject to waste or duplication. For example, most institutions have set up evaluation procedures for computer hardware and software because requests have become ubiquitous.

Safety Officer.—Common sense, and especially insurance carriers, now demand stringent electrical, fire, radiation, and other forms of safety requirements. The safety officer will want to review the specifications of the proposed instrument and will need to be assured that it complies with such codes.

Final Approving Officer.—This may be the president of the institution when very large purchases are involved, or designate in other matters. This person will need the approval of all other reviewers before he or she signs off.

Purchasing Officer.—This person ultimately will let the order be sent to the vendor. They can only act as effectively as the instructions they are given. They may also be subject to certain purchasing requirements. For example, government agencies may have specific requirements to "sole source" a particular item or, paradoxically, to allow competitive bidding. Therefore, your particular request must fit in with these requirements.

Appendix
Biomedical Engineering Literature

COMPUTERIZED ENGINEERING INDEX

COMPENDEX (Computer data base of technical literature in the engineering sciences, including biomedical engineering)
Engineering Index Inc., New York, NY

PERIODICALS

ADVANCES IN BIOTECHNOLOGICAL PROCESSES
Alan R Liss, New York, NY

ANNALS OF BIOMEDICAL ENGINEERING
Pergamon Press, Elmsford, NY

APPLIED BIOCHEMISTRY AND BIOTECHNOLOGY
Humana Press, Clifton, NJ

APPLIED MATHEMATICS AND COMPUTATION
Elsevier Science Publishing, New York, NY

AUSTRALASIAN PHYSICAL & ENGINEERING SCIENCES IN MEDI-
CINE
Australian College of Physical Sciences in Medicine, Melbourne, Aus-
tralia

AUTOMEDICA
Gordon and Breach Science Publishers, London, England

BIOENGINEERING ABSTRACTS
Engineering Information, New York, NY

BIOMEDICAL ENGINEERING AND COMPUTATION SERIES
Harwood Academic Publishers, New York, NY

BIOMEDICAL SCIENCES INSTRUMENTATION
Instrument Society of America, Pittsburgh, PA

BIOMEDIZINISCHE TECHNIK (BIOMEDICAL ENGINEERING)
German Association on Bio-Medical Enginering, Berlin, West Ger-
many

BIOPHYSICS AND BIOENGINEERING SERIES
Academic Press, New York, NY

BIOTECHNOLOGY AND BIOENGINEERING SYMPOSIUM
John Wiley & Sons, New York, NY

DIRECTORY OF BIOMEDICAL ENGINEERS
Alliance for Engineering in Medicine and Biology, Bethesda, MD

ENGINEERING IN MEDICINE
Mechanical Engineering Publications, Suffolk, England

IEEE ENGINEERING IN MEDICINE AND BIOLOGY MAGAZINE:
THE QUARTERLY MAGAZINE OF THE ENGINEERING IN MEDI-
CINE AND BIOLOGY SOCIETY
Institute of Electrical and Electronics Engineers, New York, NY

IEEE TRANSACTIONS ON BIOMEDICAL ENGINEERING
Institute of Electrical and Electronics Engineers, New York, NY

IYO DENSHI TO SETAI KOGAKU (JAPANESE JOURNAL OF MEDI-
CAL ELECTRONICS AND BIOLOGICAL ENGINEERING)
(Text in Japanese; summaries in English)
Japan Society of Medical Electronics and Biological Engineering, Co-
rona Publishing Co, Tokyo, Japan

JOURNAL OF BIOMEDICAL ENGINEERING
(Biological Engineering Society) Betterworth Scientific Ltd, Surrey, England

JOURNAL OF BIOMEDICAL MATERIALS RESEARCH
(Society for Biomaterials) John Wiley & Sons, New York, NY

JOURNAL OF CLINICAL ENGINEERING
Quest Publishing Co, Brea, CA

JOURNAL OF MEDICAL ENGINEERING & TECHNOLOGY
Taylor & Francis Ltd, Hants, England

JOURNAL OF MEDICAL ENGINEERING AND TECHNOLOGY
United Trade Press, London, England

MEDICAL & BIOLOGICAL ENGINEERING & COMPUTING
(Text in English, French and German)
International Federation for Medical Electronics and Biological Engi-
neering, Peter Peregrinus Ltd, Herts, England

MEDICAL INSTRUMENTATION
Association for the Advancement of Medical Instrumentation, Arling-
ton, VA

MEDICAL PROGRESS THROUGH TECHNOLOGY
Springer-Verlag, New York, NY

MEDICAL RESEARCH ENGINEERING
Medical-Research-Technology, Little Falls, NJ

NEWSLETTER OF BIOMEDICAL SAFETY AND STANDARDS
Quest Publishing, Brea, CA

PHYSICAL TECHNIQUES IN MEDICINE
John Wiley & Sons, New York, NY

PROGRESS IN BIOMEDICAL ENGINEERING
Elsevier, Amsterdam and New York, NY

T.I.T. JOURNAL OF LIFE SCIENCES
Tower International Technomedical Institute, Philadelphia, PA

General References

Brown JHU, Jacobs JE, Stark L (eds): *Biomedical Engineering.* Philadelphia, FA Davis Co, 1971.

Cromwell L, Arditti M, Weibell FJ, et al: *Medical Instrumentation for Health Care.* Englewood Cliffs, NJ, Prentice-Hall, 1976.

Cromwell L, Weibell FJ, Pfeiffer EA, et al: *Biomedical Instrumentation and Measurements.* Englewood Cliffs, NJ, Prentice-Hall, 1973.

Geddes LA, Baker LE: *Principles of Applied Biomedical Instrumentation,* ed 2. New York, John Wiley & Sons, 1975.

Ray CD (ed): *Medical Engineering.* Chicago, Year Book Medical Publishers, 1974.

Stacy RW: *Biological and Medical Electronics.* New York, McGraw-Hill Book Co, 1960.

Strong P: *Biophysical Measurements.* Beaverton, Ore, Tektronix, 1970. (Currently available through Spacelabs, Chatsworth, Calif.)

Yanof HM: *Biomedical Electronics,* ed 2. Philadelphia, FA Davis Co, 1972.

Further Reading

CHAPTER 1

1. Cromwell L, Arditti M, Weibell FJ, et al: The fundamentals of electricity applied to medicine, in *Medical Instrumentation for Health Care*. Englewood Cliffs, NJ, Prentice-Hall, 1976, chap 3, pp 17–65.
2. Devey GB, Montgomery LH: Electrical hazards and safety in the hospital laboratory and patient settings, in Ray CD (ed): *Medical Engineering*. Chicago, Year Book Medical Publishers, 1974, pp 1090–1096.
3. Geddes LA: Electrical hazards, in *Cardiovascular Devices and Their Application*. New York, John Wiley & Sons, 1984, pp 350–384.
4. Ray CD: Principles of electricity and electronics, in Ray CD (ed): *Medical Engineering*. Chicago, Year Book Medical Publishers, 1974, pp 861–892.
5. *Safety Clinic 1 and 2*. Chicago, Joint Commission on the Accreditation of Hospitals, 1981.
6. Steere NV (ed): Handbook of laboratory safety, ed 2. Boca Raton, Fla, CRC Press, 1971.
7. Strong P: Grounding safety, in *Biophysical Measurements*. Beaverton, Ore, Tektronix, 1972, pp 249–268. (Currently available through Spacelabs, Chatsworth, Calif.)

CHAPTER 2

1. Attinger EO, Anne A, McDonald DA: Use of Fourier series for the analysis of biological signals. *Biophys J* 1966; 6:291–304.

2. Geddes LA, Baker LE: Criteria for the faithful reproduction of an event, in *Principles of Applied Biomedical Instrumentation*. New York, John Wiley & Sons, 1968 , chap 14, pp 446–467.
3. Glantz SA: Fourier analysis, spectra, and filters. University of California Press, Berkeley, 1979, chap 6, pp 218–291.
4. Stacy RW: The theory of measurement, in *Biological and Medical Electronics*. New York, McGraw-Hill Book Co, 1960, chap 2, pp 8–26.
5. Strong P: Physiology and generation of biomedical potentials within man, in *Biophysical Measurements*. Beaverton, Ore, Tektronix, 1970, sec 1. (Currently available through Spacelabs, Chatsworth, Calif.)

CHAPTER 3

1. Carmines EG, Zeiler RA: Reliability and validity assessment, in Sullivan JL (series ed): *Quantitative Applications in the Social Sciences*. Sage, Beverly Hills, Calif, Sage University Papers, 1980.
2. Cembrowski GS: Mathematical aspects of laboratory medicine, in Ingram D, Bloch RF (eds): *Mathematical Methods in Medicine*. New York, John Wiley & Sons, 1984, pp 273–306.
3. Cobbold RSC: Biomedical measurement systems, in Ray CD (ed): *Medical Engineering*, Chicago, Year Book Medical Publishers, 1974, chap 15, pp 126–170.
4. Stacy RW: The theory of measurement, in *Biological and Medical Electronics*. New York, McGraw-Hill Book Co, 1960, chap 2, pp 8–26.
5. Yanof HM: The measurement of voltage and current, in *Biomedical Electronics*, ed 2. Philadelphia, FA Davis Co, 1972, chap 3, pp 49–64.

CHAPTER 4

1. Stacy RW: Instrumentation as a science, in *Biological and Medical Electronics*. New York, McGraw-Hill Book Co, 1960, chap 1, pp 1–7.
2. Trimmer JD: The basis for a science of instrumentology. *Science* 1953; 118:461–465.

CHAPTER 5

1. Cobbold RSC: Biomedical measurement systems, in Ray CD (ed): *Medical Engineering*. Chicago, Year Book Medical Publishers, 1974, chap 15, pp 126–170.
2. Geddes LA: Blood pressure and its direct measurement, in *Cardiovascular Devices and Their Application*. New York, John Wiley & Sons, 1984, chap 2, pp 63–99.

3. Geddes LA, Baker LE: *Principles of Applied Biomedical Instrumentation*, ed 2. New York, John Wiley & Sons, 1975.
4. *Practical Strain Gauge Measurements—Application Note 290–1*. Palo Alto, Calif, Hewlett Packard Company, 1972.
5. Offner F: Bioelectric potentials—their source, recording and significance. *IEEE Trans Biomed Engr* 1984; BME-31:863–868.
6. Stacy RW: Instrumentation as a science, in *Biological and Medical Electronics*. New York, McGraw-Hill Book Co, 1960, chap 1, pp 1–7.
7. Strong P: Electrodes, in *Biophysical Measurements*. Beaverton, Ore, Tektronix, 1972, chap 16, pp 219–248.
8. Strong P: Transducers-transducer systems, in *Biophysical Measurements*. Beaverton, Ore, Tektronix, 1972, chap 18, pp 269–291.
9. Wagner Jr HN: Instrumentation, radiopharmaceuticals and dosimetry, in Berman DS, Mason DT (eds): *Clinical Nuclear Cardiology*. New York, Grune & Stratton, 1981, chap 2, pp 28–48.
10. Weyman AE: Physical principles of ultrasound, in *Cross-sectional Echocardiography*. Philadelphia, Lea & Febiger, 1982, chap 1, pp 3–30.

CHAPTER 6

1. Jung WG: *IC Op-Amp Cookbook*, ed 2. Indianapolis, HW Sams, 1980.
2. Strong P: Amplifiers, in *Biophysical Measurements*. Beaverton, Ore, Tektronix, 1972, chap 19, pp 293–318.
3. Strong P: Signal processors—operational amplifiers, in *Biophysical Measurements*. Beaverton, Ore, Tektronix, 1972, chap 20, pp 319–336.

CHAPTER 7

1. Strong P: Oscilloscopes, in *Biophysical Measurements*. Beaverton, Ore, Tektronix, 1972, chap 21, pp 337–360.
2. Strong P: Graphics recorders, in *Biophysical Measurements*. Beaverton, Ore, Tektronix, 1972, chap 25, pp 399–412.
3. Yanof HM: The output signal and what to do with it, in *Biomedical Electronics*, ed 2. Philadelphia, FA Davis Co, 1972, chap 10, pp 215–225.

CHAPTER 8

1. Cromwell L, Arditti M, Weibell FJ, et al: Computers in health care, in *Medical Instrumentation for Health Care*. Englewood Cliffs, NJ, Prentice-Hall, 1976, chap 19, pp 348–362.
2. Foster CC: The sampling theorem, in *Real Time Programming*. Reading, Pa, Addison-Wesley Co, 1981, chap 6, pp 77–85.
3. Sheldon K (ed): Theme—mass storage. *Byte* 1986; 11:158–249.

CHAPTER 9

1. Frequency response of liquid-filled pressure recording systems, in *Application Notes,* vol 1, no 5. Mahwah, New Jersey, Irex Medical Systems, 1974.
2. Manktelow RT, Baird RJ: A practical approach to accurate pressure measurements. *J Thorac Cardiovasc Surg* 1969; 58:122–127.
3. Webster JG: Reducing motion artifacts and interference in biopotential recording. *IEEE Trans Biomed Engr* 1984; 31:823–826.
4. Wolbarsht ML, Spekreijse H: Interference and noise in biological instrumentation, in Levine SN (ed): *Advances in Biomedical Engineering and Medical Physics.* New York, John Wiley & Sons, 1968, vol 2, pp 205–242.

CHAPTER 10

1. Cromwell L, Arditti M, Weibell FJ, et al: Care and use of electronic equipment, in *Medical Instrumentation for Health Care.* Englewood Cliffs, NJ, Prentice-Hall, 1976, chap 10, pp 363–375.
2. Stacy RW: Troubleshooting instruments, in *Biological and Medical Electronics.* New York, McGraw-Hill Book Co, 1960, chap 9, pp 229–250.

Index